Comments on *Heart Health at youɪ*

'I enjoyed reading it. Graham Jackson ɪs a ᴠⅽⅼ̩ _
he explains things very well for the layman.'

Dr RICHARD WRAY, Consultant Physician, Department of Cardiology,
The Conquest Hospital, St Leonards on Sea

'This edition is superb and is suitable for any patient with heart disease or
who is afraid of developing heart disease. It could prove very useful to
medical practitioners as it contains detailed ways for their patients to
modify their lifestyles so that heart disease risk is minimal.'

Dr IAN BAIRD, former Medical Spokesman, British Heart Foundation

'This is an excellent book and I struggled to find any gaps or ways to
improve it. Every household or family that has someone suffering from
heart disease should have a copy of this book, which contains answers to
many questions and much sound advice.'

Professor MIKE KIRBY, Visiting Professor Faculty of Health
and Human Sciences, University of Hertfordshire

'An excellent guide to practicalities of heart health for patients.'

Dr ANTHONY WIERZBICKI, Consultant in Chemical Pathology,
Guy's and St Thomas' NHS Foundation Trust

Comments on *Heart Health – the 'at your fingertips guide'* from readers

'He has successfully managed the difficult task of dealing with a broad
canvas of heart disorders in combination with useful advice on a healthy
lifestyle. This book is eminently readable.'

Dr IAN BAIRD, Trustee, HOPE Project,
former Medical Spokesman, British Heart Foundation

'Coronary heart disease is the biggest single killer of men and women in
this country. There is, therefore, no better time to promote good health,
and Dr Jackson's book is most welcome.'

FRANK DOBSON, former Secretary of State for Health

'An excellent resource for people seeking answers.'

LYNNE SWEENEY, Technical Advisor, The Family Heart Association

'A very readable book.'

AZMINA GOVINDJI, Consultant Nutritionist and Dietitian

'I believe the author has got the balance right between being too technical and over-simplification. The book leaves the reader reassured that the questions have been answered by a person at the top of his particular field of work. I genuinely believe I am the better for having read this book.'

T Moody, Hitchin, Herts

'There were always questions that I had failed to ask but with the new book there is so far nothing to which, as a patient, I have been unable to find an answer.'

GEOFFREY SEGROVE, Chalfont St Peter, Bucks

'Your book has given me more support than any doctor, hospital or support group. I found it very informative and it answered a lot of questions I forgot to ask when talking to the doctor.'

GWYNETH FENTON, London

'I found great comfort and an insight into my illness after reading this book.'

D BRADLEY, Falkirk

'Of the books we have consulted, we have found yours the more accessible and helpful.'

V BUTTERS, Coventry

'I always keep the book to hand and dip into it when I want to know something. The book is well written, and very straightforward and understandable and I will gladly recommend this book to anyone who has a heart problem.'

IAN GOLDING, Darlington

'Graham Jackson takes the reader on a voyage of discovery and explanation in his clearly written and good humoured text, which should allay fear through awareness of what heart disease is all about.'

Professor BRIAN L PENTECOST MD FRCP, former Medical Director
of the British Heart Foundation

Reviews of *Heart Health – the 'at your fingertips guide'*

'... a veritable *vade mecum* of its subject, written for patients and the sort of book that I could have done with some 20 years ago.'

Cardiology News

'Busy doctors, or dissatisfied heart patients, couldn't do better than invest in Dr Jackson's latest book *Heart Health at your fingertips*. It contains 260 pages devoted to questions that patients ask and answers the doctor wishes he had given if only he'd had the time to think how best to put them.'

Dr THOMAS STUTTAFORD, *The Times*

'Those readers who want to know more about the various treatments for heart disease will be much enlightened.'

Dr James Le Fanu, *The Daily Telegraph*

'One of the most straightforward and helpful books on heart disease that I have ever read ... Dr Jackson isn't lecturing me, but rather he is sitting alongside me, answering my questions in a way that makes sense to me.'

Heart News

'Visits to the surgery or the hospital are often not the best time or setting for patients to receive answers to questions or concerns. Those who have experienced this frustration will find Dr Jackson's book a most useful and informative resource. Heart health at your fingertips comes highly recommended.'

The Family Heart Digest

'Here's a book you might want to have to hand for all those questions you would like to ask but don't know where or who to consult. Dr Jackson gives straightforward advice together with all the latest information about coronary heart disease.'

In Balance magazine

'The medical expertise of Consultant Cardiologist Dr Graham Jackson is now available to people all over the UK.'

People, Guy's and St Thomas' Hospitals magazine

'The joy of this book is that it is not a medical textbook but a book giving information about the practical problems of heart disease and its prevention or treatment. It is easy reading, dip in and out, with a format of questions and answers – questions we all want to ask followed by well thought out answers. Highly recommended.'

Heart Digest

'I would recommend this book to any patient or member of the general public expressing an interest in keeping their heart healthy.'

British Journal of Cardiology

'I found the book easy to read, and would recommend it, especially in today's climate with the national emphasis on coronary heart disease.'

The Pharmaceutical Journal

Heart health
Answers at your fingertips

FOURTH EDITION

Graham Jackson FESC, FACC, FRCP

Honorary Consultant Cardiologist,
Guy's and St Thomas' Hospital Trust,
St Thomas' Hospital, London SE1

CLASS PUBLISHING · LONDON

Printing history
First published 1998; Second edition 2000; Third edition 2004; Fourth edition 2009

The author and publisher welcome feedback from the users of this book. Please contact the publisher.

Class Publishing Ltd, Barb House, Barb Mews, London W6 7PA, UK
Telephone: 020 7371 2119 [International +4420]
Fax: 020 7371 2878
Email: post@class.co.uk
Visit our website – www.class.co.uk

The information presented in this book is accurate and current to the best of the author's knowledge. The author and publisher, however, make no guarantee as to, and assume no responsibility for, the correctness, sufficiency or completeness of such information or recommendation. The reader is advised to consult a doctor regarding all aspects of individual healthcare.

A CIP catalogue record for this book is available from the British Library

ISBN 1 85959 157 4

10 9 8 7 6 5 4 3 2 1

Previous editions edited by Michèle Clarke

This edition edited by Caroline Sheldrick

Cartoons by Linda Moore

Illustrations by David Woodroffe

Designed and typeset by Martin Bristow

Printed and bound in Finland by WS Bookwell, Juva

Contents

LIFESTYLE HINTS

Dedication
For Maggie, Keira and Matthew

Acknowledgements

It would have been impossible to write this book without the help of Richard Warner and the team at Class. They helped me write plain English and were supportive when it all seemed overwhelming. I am grateful to Ronnie Corbett for providing such a warm foreword. Dr Richard Wray, Dr Ian Baird, Tony Wierzbicki and Mike Kirby reviewed the text and provided extremely helpful suggestions and identified areas that I had not made clear or helpful. Azmina Govinda, with her expert knowledge as a consultant nutritionist, has made sure that the sections on diet and lifestyle make sense. I would like to thank Linda Moore for the delightful cartoons and David Woodroffe for the clear illustrations. I need to acknowledge all my patients who have gladly provided most of the questions and have in turn helped me answer them I hope in a way that is helpful and clear.

Foreword

by **Ronnie Corbett** OBE
Actor and comedian

Anne and I were having a short break, perhaps six or seven days in New York, early autumn, and staying at the wondrously delightful and cosy hotel called The Carlyle. The Carlyle famous for its association with the piano entertainer Bobby Short, and of course the same Carlyle as Woody Allen very often has his jam sessions on the clarinet. It is really like home. Curiously enough on our most recent visit we bumped into Elaine Stritch, and she actually lives there, upstairs, as a permanent home.

Anyway, Anne and I were having this break in a chilly New York, wind factor very high, very noticeable in the geometric style in which central New York is laid out. We were walking all over the place, shopping here and there; actually in truth I was looking for a particular shop that sells Borsalino hats, just passing the time, but sort of wasting it, and making a rather arduous trip for Anne. This is the first time this sort of effort had seemed arduous to her, and she and I were both aware that when she got home it would be worth having it checked out. This she did, and so we met for the first time Dr Graham Jackson, and within days he had suggested she went to Mr Christopher Blauth at the London Bridge Hospital, where she probably had a major heart operation. It was in fact extremely major, because it was an aortic valve transplant.

Heart features in my family a bit, because my dad died, prematurely really, at the age of 75 playing his second round of golf in the week. He was an extremely well controlled diabetic and had been for 40 years, and he had this problem which was then called angina, but little was known of it really by today's standard, and he dropped dead playing the fifteenth hole, as I say, and never came home for his tea. A terrible shock for us all, but mainly for my mum, who was looking out of the window with his high tea prepared, as she had done all their lives together. So she was lost, completely lost. My mother by contrast lived to the age of 93, with a very strong heart indeed, and no need to diet or campaign in the same way that my dear dad had to.

So really heart features strongly in our lives, and I in the shadow of Anne's care have come under Graham's eagle eye and tried to watch my weight, unsuccessfully of course, but fortunately my diet of fish and fruit, and not too much drink, kind of helps me.

So from the circuitous route I have been asked by Graham to write the foreword to this book. I've never done such a thing before; this is my first attempt and I will perhaps get eight out of ten for it. Anyway, best wishes with the book. I have enjoyed the previous ones, and I hope you enjoy this one.

Kind regards
Yours aye

Preface to the fourth edition

Since the third edition, more progress has been made in preventing coronary artery disease. New guidelines and targets have been introduced as a result of continuing research. Fewer men and women are dying of heart disease but as we live longer, keeping active and healthy becomes increasingly important. The benefits of lowering cholesterol and blood pressure and stopping smoking are unfortunately offset by increasing incidence of obesity and diabetes as well as physical inactivity, so all aspects of heart health need attention: not just one or two.

Most heart attacks, 90% in fact, are caused by factors we can do something about. This fourth edition shows you how to help yourself as well as explaining the medical and surgical treatments on offer. We do not have all the answers, but we have a lot we can work on. Once more, to the many who have contacted me – thank you for your comments and helpful suggestions.

Introduction

This book is principally about your heart: how to keep it strong or, if it has been weakened in some way, how to make it as strong as possible. The major cause of weakening of your heart is called coronary artery disease (CAD). The coronary arteries are those arteries which feed the heart itself. They arise from the main artery leaving the heart, the aorta, and run around the outside of the heart, sending many branches into the heart's muscle. They deliver oxygen and energy so that the heart can do its job of pumping blood around the body. If the coronary arteries become narrowed, the blood supply to the heart will be restricted. The result is that when the heart needs to beat faster (such as when you are walking up a hill), your heart will be starved of energy and begin to complain, usually by causing chest pain (known as angina). If a coronary artery blocks completely, there will a sudden loss of blood to a portion of heart muscle, chemicals build up, you will experience severe pain and a heart attack occurs as part of the muscle stops working. If a big coronary artery blocks, the heart attack will be large; if a small artery is blocked, there will only be a small loss of muscle.

Coronary disease is our greatest medical enemy and as much a threat to women as to men. Women may think of it as a man's disease, but it is an equal opportunity killer with no respect for sex, race or religion. Coronary heart disease kills nearly 117 000 men and women in the UK each year, and in America 450 000 adults die each year of coronary artery disease; over one-third of these are women. This means that an average of 320 people a day (or one person every four-and-a half minutes) die from coronary artery disease in the UK. Women may be more afraid of breast cancer but it is more than five times as likely that they will die from the consequences of heart disease. It is so common that one in three adults of both sexes over 65 years of age has some form of heart disease.

The cost of coronary disease affects both you personally (causing stress and uncertainty, and affecting social and family life) and the community, with the National Health Service bill for heart disease per year estimated to be over 3500 million pounds. The key to preventing coronary disease happening to you is to understand the causes, and to know how to reduce the chances of it developing. It is never too late to act for yourself and your family.

In this book you will discover how the heart works and how coronary artery disease develops. The emphasis is on prevention; both prevention before heart problems occur, which is called primary prevention, and prevention after you have been diagnosed as having coronary disease, which is called secondary prevention. Both are important – when you have a disease, you want to stop it getting worse, and when you have no evidence of disease, you want to keep it that way. Sections of this book are concerned with diet, exercise, smoking and blood pressure control, and the importance of reducing your risk factors for coronary disease. A risk factor is something that increases your likelihood of developing a disease, and an easy example of this is cigarette smoking. Smokers have more coronary disease than non-smokers, and smokers who quit reduce their risk after a period of 4–5 years to the same as non-smokers. Advice is given on risk factors and how to minimise your risk.

The consequences of coronary artery disease are discussed, with advice on treatments available, and how you can help yourself. Doctors need to have good evidence that a form of treatment is effective; this is known as 'evidence-based medicine'. It is important that you understand the benefits and risks of any therapy recommended to you: be fully informed and ask questions – it's your heart after all! Just as I must provide evidence that medical treatments are effective, you must ask for similar evidence from unconventional treatments that you may have read about: do not believe all you are told – ask for the evidence. Remember, however, that the quality of evidence can vary. It is easy to be convinced, on the basis of personal experience or that of a close friend or relative, that the disease has been 'cured'. It is unfortunately easy to be deluded as most diseases are very variable and impressions of a 'cure' may be misguided. The only way to establish genuine benefit is from scientific trials. These try to remove chance or, put another way, remove the possibility that you would have got better anyway.

There are sections on angina, heart attacks, drugs and bypass surgery; and the role of angioplasty (balloon treatment) and the placement of a stent (an expandable metal cage) to hold arteries open, is covered in detail.

This is not a medical textbook but a book giving information about the practical problems of coronary artery disease and its prevention or treatment. It deals with the commonest questions asked and tries to answer in the clearest way. Not all questions have easy answers so, where there are grey areas, these are discussed in an attempt to clarify what, for doctors as well as patients, can be a difficult subject.

Coronary artery disease can be thought of as a series of keys – the first key is the key to prevention; the second, the key to early recognition of warning symptoms; the third, the key to the correct treatment, and the fourth, the key to preventing it happening again. This book is about finding the keys, and information is vital for finding them all. Armed with this book, you will be in a good position to do so.

HOW TO USE THIS BOOK

If you do not understand the terms used, check in the glossary at the back. The book is written in a way that allows you to dip into it, rather than read it from cover to cover. It's a good idea to read Chapter 1 before any other, just to be sure that you understand how the heart works. With a good background, the rest is easier to follow.

You may want to know about drug treatment for angina (see the section *Treatment* in Chapter 3) but it's best to see how it compares with other treatments in order to get a broader view and to see what options are available. The same applies to heart attack patients or their relatives – read around the subject to get a better perspective.

QUESTIONS FOR YOUR DOCTOR OR PRACTICE NURSE

Books like this try to answer as many questions as possible, but they should encourage you to ask your doctor questions also. No one ever remembers to ask questions in the surgery. Write your questions down before you visit the surgery, making a list like a shopping list. If your doctor cannot answer them, write to me (at the publisher's address at the beginning of this book) and I will try to answer them for you.

FINALLY

- Don't be afraid of heart disease.
- Learn about it to understand it.
- Do your best to prevent it.
- Learn to cope with it.
- Remember, despite suffering heart problems, most people lead full and active lives as a result of modern treatments.

1 | How your heart works

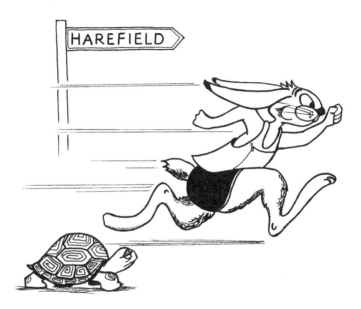

Your heart is a pump made of muscle which pushes blood through your arteries to all organs of your body. The body needs oxygen and energy to work normally and blood is the delivery system. Blood picks up its oxygen in the lungs and becomes bright red as a result. After it gives up its oxygen, blood takes carbon dioxide and waste products for elimination to the lungs, liver and kidneys in the veins, where it is a now a dark red colour. Your heart muscle needs oxygen and energy and this is obtained from the blood through the coronary arteries. Disease of the coronary arteries is the commonest cause of death and disability in the western world because it stops the heart – the body's engine – doing its job properly.

ANATOMY OF THE HEART

What is the heart?

The heart is a muscular pump but it is a very sophisticated one. It is made of muscle different from the sort that moves your arms and legs. Heart muscle is particularly strong as it has to cope with the physical and emotional stresses of normal daily life and, of course, it never takes a rest (you hope!). It beats on average 100 000 times every 24 hours and pumps out between 5 and 20 litres of blood (1 litre equals just under 2 pints) every minute, depending on your body's needs – more when you are being active than when you are resting. Every organ in the body needs oxygen to function normally and efficiently. Fresh blood in the arteries delivers oxygen and energy to your body tissues and then, when it has given up its energy supply, blood carries away in the veins unwanted waste products including carbon dioxide. The heart is the engine that pumps the blood around; normally it is the size of a clenched fist.

Can you tell me what the coronary arteries are?

These are the tubes or vessels that supply your heart muscle with the oxygen and energy that it needs to pump efficiently. The vessels that carry the oxygen round the body are called arteries. Coronary arteries* are tough tubes able to cope with the pressure pumped out by the heart. They are often confused with veins, such as those that we see on the back of the hand or on the legs (usually blue). Veins bring used-up blood back to the heart. They are thinner than arteries and do not work or cope with high pressure in the same way as arteries do.

Think of your coronary arteries like the branches of a big tree with a main trunk branching out into smaller and smaller branches and

*There is a glossary on page 297 to help you with unfamiliar terms.

twigs. There are three important coronary arteries with many branches. There is a left coronary artery which divides into two large branches, and a right coronary artery which is usually one big vessel (see Figure 1.1). The coronary arteries arise from the main artery leaving your heart (the *aorta*), beginning just above the aortic valve (see question below). The most important coronary artery is the left

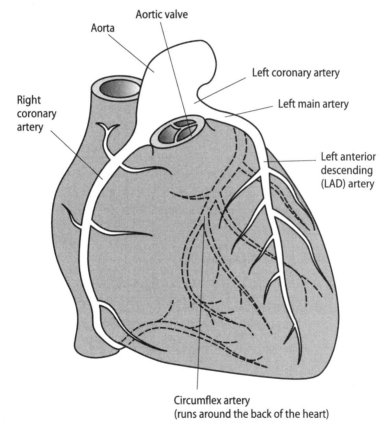

Figure 1.1 The coronary arteries surround the heart muscle and send branches into the muscle, delivering blood containing oxygen. They start from the aorta just above the aortic valve. Dotted lines indicate the arteries running around the back of the heart.

main stem, which controls both branches of the left coronary artery and, as a result, most of the blood supply to your heart muscle.

The coronary arteries start at about 3–4 mm in size (like a thin straw) and as they feed the muscle they divide to reach all the layers of muscle. They run around the outside of the heart, sending their branches inwards.

What happens when things go wrong with the coronary arteries?

The inner lining of your arteries is called the endothelium (pro-nounced 'en-doe-thee-li-um') which is a smooth surface allowing the blood to flow easily. If the endothelium becomes damaged, the tube becomes narrower, and the blood flow becomes turbulent with a chance of clots forming. Think of the artery as a roadway with a new road surface (the endothelium) – now imagine what happens to traffic flow if potholes are allowed to develop and road works cone off one or two lanes or humps are introduced – drive too fast and you will come a cropper! Your endothelium can become damaged by:

- cigarette smoking;

- poorly treated high blood pressure; and

- a high level of cholesterol in your blood, causing localised deposits of fatty material ('road humps').

Narrowed coronary arteries can cause:

- angina;

- heart attack: the medical term for this is *myocardial* (heart muscle) *infarction* (death of part of the heart muscle) (see Chapter 4);

- irregular heartbeats (some types of palpitations, see Chapter 6); and heart failure (where your muscle becomes weak, see Chapter 5).

What is the aorta?

The aorta is the main artery leaving your heart. It sends blood to your head and then curves over to run down your chest along the spine. It passes along the back of your stomach, and at the top of the legs it divides into the big arteries which send branches down to your feet. Arteries branch off the aorta supplying arms, legs and all the important organs, such as the kidneys and liver.

What are the valves?

The valves control the flow of blood into and out of your heart. They open and shut just like a tap being turned on and off. When working normally, they act as one-way valves. The valves are on the inside of your heart, whereas the coronary arteries are on the outside. There are four valves – the aortic, mitral, pulmonary and tricuspid. Look at Figure 1.2 and see the sequence of events.

1. Blood returns to your heart through the veins. It has given up its oxygen to your brain, kidneys and muscle. It comes from the head region in a big vein called the *superior* (from the top of the body) *vena cava*, and from the lower body in a big vein called the *inferior vena cava*. It collects in a chamber called the right *atrium*.

2. The tricuspid valve separates this collecting chamber from the right ventricle, which is part of your muscle pump. (*Ventricle* is the medical word for pump.) You will notice the use of the word 'right' at this stage. This is because your heart is divided into two sides. The right side (on your right) collects used-up blood and passes it to your lungs to pick up oxygen, and the left collects oxygen-rich blood from the lungs and pumps it round the body. The muscle pump on the left is called the left ventricle. This is the most important part of the heart and the one that is most often damaged in a heart attack.

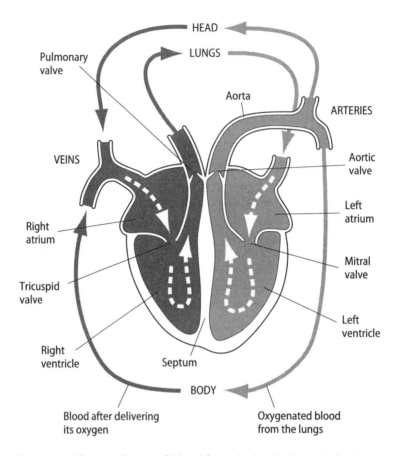

Figure 1.2 The circulation of blood from the body through the heart to the lungs. From the lungs the blood containing oxygen returns to the heart and circulates to the rest of the body. The atria are the collecting chambers; the ventricles are the muscle pump.

③ On the left side of your heart, blood leaving the lungs has been collecting in the left atrium. Blood therefore collects in the right atrium and left atrium at the same time. Separating the left atrium from the left ventricle is the *mitral valve*. The mitral valve opens at the same time as the tricuspid valve so that blood enters the right and left ventricles almost simultaneously.

4 Both the right ventricle and left ventricle contract at the same time. As the pressure builds up, the force closes the tricuspid and mitral valves (preventing any leaking backwards) and opens the *pulmonary* and *aortic valves*. Blood is ejected through the pulmonary valve to your lungs, and the aortic valve to your body. When the pump has emptied, the pressure drops, the pulmonary and aortic valves close, and the tricuspid and mitral valves open again; the cycle is then repeated.

What keeps the right and left heart apart?

The muscle that divides your heart is called the *septum*. Between the right and left atrium, it is known as the atrial septum, and between the ventricles, the ventricular septum. When a hole occurs in your heart, we call it a defect. If it is between the atria (plural of atrium), it is known as an *atrial septal defect* (ASD) and if it is between the ventricles, it is a *ventricular septal defect* (VSD).

HOW YOUR HEART WORKS

When I asked my doctor how my heart works, he said that it would take too long to explain! Can you tell me simply how the normal heart works?

The healthy normal heart is made up of strong muscle and four valves in full working order. It gets its oxygen from blood supplied by the coronary arteries. It is controlled by an electric circuit which tells it when to beat and how fast to beat. The medical term for contraction of your heart pump (that is, when the heart beats, felt as the pulse) is *systole*, and when the heart relaxes (between the beats or pulse), *diastole*.

The nurse at our practice runs a clinic to test blood pressures.
What is blood pressure exactly and why is it so important?

We all need a blood pressure to keep our blood flowing round our bodies. It is the pressure of the blood in the arteries that is needed for delivering oxygen and food where it is needed and taking away waste products to the kidneys and liver.

Blood pressure has two terms applied to it – systolic and diastolic. The *systolic pressure* is the top (highest) pressure and is at its maximum following each heartbeat. The bottom (lowest) pressure (*diastolic pressure*) is the lowest recording between heartbeats when your heart is resting. You might see, for example, 120 (systolic)/80 (diastolic) given as millimetres of mercury and, as mercury's symbol is Hg, you will see 120/80 mmHg, or 120/80 for short. Mercury is simply a visible liquid used to show the difference between liquid and pressure. When pressure is increased, the mercury is pushed up the scale of the blood pressure machine (the *sphygmomanometer*; see **Measurement of blood pressure** in Chapter 2) and readings can be taken in millimetres or mm for short. The mercury sphygmomanometer is being phased out in some countries including the UK and being replaced by electronic machines. This development is regrettable as not all electronic machines are as accurate as the sphygmomanometer (particularly when there is an irregular heart rhythm or very high blood pressure).

I know that the heart beats automatically, but what, if anything,
keeps it going?

The heart gets its instructions rather like an electric circuit (see Figure 1.3). There is a master switch called the *sinus node* which speeds up the heart rate and slows it down depending on your body's needs. If you are feeling emotional, or running, it goes faster; if you are resting or sleeping, it goes slower.

The sinus node sends messages to a junction box (the *atrio-ventricular node* or AV node) which regulates the electric impulses

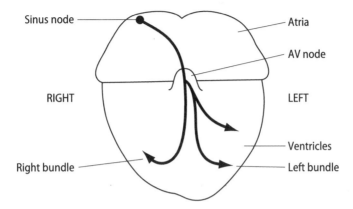

Figure 1.3 The 'electrics' of the heart.

before allowing them through into the 'wires' that supply the left heart muscle (ventricle) known as the *left bundle*, or the right ventricle known as the *right bundle*. In this way, if some problem develops so that the control switch races away, the junction box protects your heart by not allowing it to go out of control. Normal impulses start in the sinus node, and travel via the atrioventricular node to the 'bundles of wires' that supply the left or right ventricle. The right bundle is single, whilst the left bundle divides into branches (Figure 1.3).

WHAT CAN GO WRONG WITH MY HEART?

Various things can go wrong with your heart:

- a problem with the pump: the muscle might become weak (thin) or too thick (hypertrophy);

- damage to your valves: they might become narrow or develop leaks;

- your coronary arteries might become narrowed or blocked; or

- the 'electrics' might fail: they might short circuit and go too fast or too slow or alternate between fast and slow.

More than one thing can happen at once and one problem can lead to another. This book will explain that there is plenty that you can do to prevent or deal with the problems that occur.

The heart may also be faulty from birth. This condition is known as *congenital* (present at birth, by chance) *heart disease* and can occasionally be inherited (passed on from your parents through your genes).

I am 46 and sometimes feel odd sensations in my chest. Are these to do with my heart? How will I know if I have a heart problem?

The main symptoms people get are:

- chest pain;
- breathlessness;
- palpitations;
- blackouts (less commonly).

If your heart muscle weakens, then you may feel tired or 'washed out', feeling as though you have heavy legs or thinking everything is an effort. Of course, there may be other causes for these symptoms and your doctor will be able to sort them out.

What is the commonest heart problem for me to watch out for?

Coronary artery disease (hardening or narrowing of the arteries to the heart) is the most common problem. The next chapters deal with each condition in turn, describing what the problem is and what treatment is available.

What is the pericardium?

The heart is covered by a thin, silky-smooth lining called the pericardium (*peri-car-dee-um*). It is known as the *pericardial sac.*

Sometimes it becomes inflamed and, instead of being silky, it becomes more like sandpaper and, if the heart rubs against it, it will be painful. Fluid can accumulate in the sac compressing the heart (*pericardial effusion*) leading to breathlessness and a low blood pressure. If necessary, the fluid can be removed under a local anaesthetic to give instant relief. Inflammation of the pericardium is known as *pericarditis*.

2 | Coronary heart disease

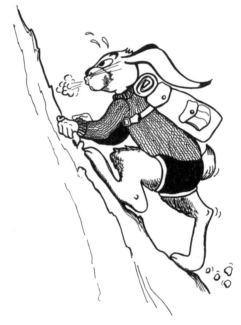

Coronary artery disease is caused by a hardening or narrowing of the arteries to your heart. The medical term is *atheroma* or *atherosclerosis*. Patches of the inner lining of the arteries become furred up from a mixture of fat, cholesterol and cells deposited in the wall. Veins, unlike arteries, do not 'fur up' unless they are asked to do the work of arteries, for example after a bypass operation (see **Bypass surgery** in Chapter 3). If you think of an artery as a three-lane motorway, the narrowed part of the artery is like a lane of the motorway being coned off; the flow of blood is restricted a bit like the traffic is slowed down as it tries to filter into the lanes that are open. The patches of narrowing are called *plaque* (pronounced 'plack'), so you may hear doctors refer to *atheromatous plaque* or plaque disease. Plaque may cause a progressive narrowing of your arteries, restricting blood flow and causing angina (see Chapter 3), or it may rupture or tear causing clots to form, which totally block the artery, and this can lead to a heart attack.

The major causes of atheroma developing are:

- raised cholesterol level;

- cigarette smoking; and

- high blood pressure.

Usually symptoms develop leading to a diagnosis of angina, heart attack or heart failure. Occasionally, the first evidence may be when someone dies suddenly from a heart attack, but there is usually a warning and it is important to understand what the warning signs are.

There are some factors in a person's life called *risk factors*. People with risk factors have an increased chance of developing a particular condition. For example, working with asbestos or down a coalmine increases the chance (or risk) of developing lung disease, and is thus considered a risk factor. Risk factors for coronary artery disease can be divided into those that can be avoided and those that can not (see Table 2.1). Avoidable risk factors, including diabetes, account for 90% of coronary disease. Risk factors for coronary disease are like penalty

Table 2.1 Avoidable and unavoidable risk factors for heart disease

Avoidable	*Unavoidable*
Cigarette smoking	Male sex
High blood pressure	Family history
High cholesterol	Diabetes (unavoidable to some extent)
Obesity	Age (getting older)
Diabetes (avoidable in many)	
Lack of exercise	
Stress	
Low intake of fruit and vegetables	
Excess alcohol	

points on a driving licence, only they multiply rather than add up: smoking may give you 3 penalty points and high blood pressure 3 penalty points, but both risk factors at the same time may give you 9 penalty points; if you also have 3 penalty points for a high cholesterol level, then your penalty points may multiply to 27 in total.

Are there any risk factors that I can't change?

Your parents, your age and your sex may increase your risks. Your race may also bring risk: people from the Indian subcontinent have more coronary disease, African-Caribbeans less. Having a family history of heart disease, being a male and getting older means that you need to take more care. A high risk family is one in which a close female relative aged 65 years or less, or a male relative aged 55 years or less, or both, developed coronary disease.

But remember that you can lessen many of your risk factors and improve your chances of not developing heart problems.

Prevention is always the best medicine so the first part of this chapter looks at what puts you at risk of developing coronary artery disease, and then how it can be prevented or treated.

RISKS OF SMOKING

I have smoked since my teens just as my father and grandfather did. My father is still alive and my grandfather lived until he was 65. What are my risks of heart disease?

There is overwhelming evidence that smoking causes hardening of the coronary arteries as well as hardening of your arteries to the brain and legs; this hardening leads to narrowed arteries and thus poor blood flow to your heart. It also leads to chronic lung diseases as well as lung cancer, and increases your chances of developing a stomach ulcer. Whilst some people escape the consequences of cigarette smoking, the majority do not.

There is a lot of talk about the harmful effects of passive smoking. Can other people's smoke really harm me?

Smoking harms any non-smokers who are breathing in the same air as a smoker, increasing their chance of heart and lung disease. It may also cause sore red eyes, headaches and make asthma worse. This has become known as *passive smoking*. Children brought up in a household of smokers suffer more infections and disease, compared to those who live in non-smoking households.

The government gives us dire warnings about smoking but I know many people who smoke who are in their seventies or eighties. Are the statistics regarding the harmful effects of smoking really as bad as the press makes out?

Yes. Smoking causes one in five deaths in our population and at least a third of these are due to heart disease. This means that, in the UK, smoking kills over 100 000 people a year. It kills 90% of the 40 000 who die from lung cancer, 75% of the 20 000 who die from chronic lung disease such as emphysema, and 25% of the 117 000 who die each year from coronary artery disease. Smoking respects no one – it is an equal opportunity killer attacking both sexes and all races. Out of the total number of people who smoke, a quarter will die early as a result, losing an average 10–15 years of life. Worldwide, smoking kills three million people a year. This is predicted to increase to 10 million by 2025, which means that 200 million of today's children and teenagers will be killed by tobacco. Add these to today's adults and we get a staggering half a billion of the world's population being killed by tobacco – 250 million dying young (aged 35–69 years) and each person losing 20 years of expected life. Many people die only after a long disabling disease.

I have changed to a low-tar brand of cigarettes, with a filter.
Why will smoking be so harmful to me now?

Components of tobacco, such as tars, are harmful to your health but the main cause is the nicotine in cigarettes as this is an addictive drug. Nicotine increases your heart rate and blood pressure making your heart work harder, whilst at the same time narrowing the arteries. Oxygen is removed from the blood and replaced with carbon monoxide. Carbon monoxide reduces the ability of the blood to carry oxygen and, in heavy smokers, may reduce it by as much as 50%. We have all read of tragedies caused by faulty gas heaters – carbon monoxide build-up is the cause. This means that there is less energy circulating to your heart to cope with the demands that nicotine places on it. The carbon monoxide level in the blood after smoking one cigarette exceeds the legal limit for pollution allowed in industry by eight times. Low tar cigarettes are nice in theory, because it is the tar in cigarettes that causes lung cancer, but actually they make matters worse in that most low tar smokers inhale deeper and increase their carbon monoxide and nicotine blood levels.

Smoking can cause roughening of the smooth lining of your arteries (the *endothelium*) and this may lead to the development of narrowed areas in the arteries caused by fat being deposited there. Smoking lowers the good cholesterol known as the high density lipoprotein (HDL) (see the section **Risks of high cholesterol levels**) and increases the blood ingredient (*fibrinogen*) that promotes clotting. Smoking therefore not only causes hardening of your arteries but increases the chance of clots forming on the narrowed areas and thus a heart attack.

I have tried again and again to give up smoking. Are there any
'safe' cigarettes?

No. All cigarettes, 'light' or not, are just as harmful to your heart. Filters have no advantages and may actually increase the carbon monoxide inhaled. Changing to low tar/nicotine cigarettes may reduce your risk of lung cancer, but not heart disease, and it is heart disease that is the major killer.

I cannot stop smoking. Would it help if I just cut down on my smoking?

Yes, but there is no such thing as safe smoking. Smoking five cigarettes a day doubles your risk of heart disease and smoking 20 a day increases your risk by at least 10 times. Reducing the number of cigarettes smoked helps, but quitting is better.

Both my husband and I smoke one pack of cigarettes a day. I have recently read that women are as much at risk as men. Is this true?

Yes and, if anything, more so (see Figure 2.1). Women seem to be more sensitive to the effects of cigarettes, so for a similar number smoked (20 per day) you are twice as likely as your husband to develop coronary artery disease. Smoking is especially dangerous if you are on the contraceptive pill, particularly if you are aged over 35 years or

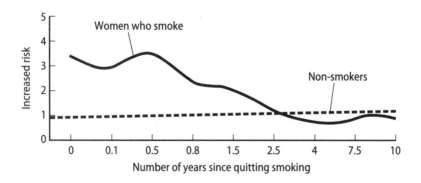

Figure 2.1 Women who smoke have almost four times as great a risk of heart attack but, three years after quitting, the risk is the same as for non-smokers. Solid line = women who smoke; dotted line = non-smokers.

have been continuously on the pill for 5 years or more (see **Women and coronary artery disease** on p. 73).

If I could stop smoking, would this do any real good?

The benefits of stopping begin quickly. By 24 hours the carbon monoxide is eliminated from the blood and the lungs begin to clear the mucus. Smell and taste improve by 48 hours. By 3 months, breathing is easier as the circulation improves, making exercise easier. By one year, the risk of a heart attack is halved, and four to five years after quitting smoking your risk of heart disease will be the same as for a non-smoker. Stopping smoking is one of the most important actions you can make – not starting is the best educational message of all (Figure 2.2). The benefit to your lungs regarding cancer takes longer – about 20 years in total, but the risk is halved by 10 years.

I am 58 and have been smoking for many years. Is it ever too late to stop?

No. The benefit to your heart is rapid and helps you, no matter what your age.

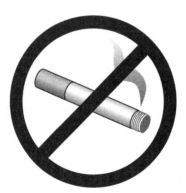

Figure 2.2 Cigarette smoking is the biggest risk factor for sudden death. The best advice is: If you smoke – QUIT; if you don't smoke – DON'T START.

My girlfriend has suggested that I change to a pipe as she is convinced that pipes and cigars are safer than cigarettes. Is this true?

Smoke from pipes and cigars contains a higher concentration of tar and nicotine compared with cigarettes, but pipe and cigar smokers usually inhale less than cigarette smokers so the risks are less, but they are still greater than in non-smokers. Cigarette smokers who switch to a pipe usually inhale the smoke automatically, thereby not significantly reducing their risks. Inhaling from a large cigar is the same as inhaling from a pack of 20 cigarettes!

Studies have shown that smokers who switch to pipes and cigars, and don't inhale, reduce their risks of lung cancer and heart disease by 50%, but the risk is still 50% higher than quitting altogether. However, by not inhaling, pipe and cigar smokers increase the risk to non-smokers from passive smoking. The best option is not to smoke at all. The principal reason pipe smokers have less risk is that they spend most of their time trying to light the pipe rather than puffing on it!

I have tried to stop smoking but always lapse. What can I do to quit smoking and avoid the temptations?

Stopping smoking is difficult but it is the biggest single improvement to your health that you, as a smoker, can make. Some people find that reading a book on quitting gives them the confidence that they need to actually stop. There are some suggestions on book titles that may be helpful in Appendix 3.

Cutting down is a help but only if your aim is to stop completely (see question above). Remember that after 3–5 years you will have your heart's health back. Here are some guidelines to help you.

- Make a list of your reasons for stopping, keep it with you and read it every day. The best reasons are:
  - it is bad for my health;
  - the cough is unpleasant;

- my clothes always smell;
- it is expensive;
- I cannot taste my food;
- non-smokers are upset by my smoking.

- Set a day to stop or take part in a sponsored 'stop' with friends or business colleagues.

- Take time for exercise, drink plenty of water and have plenty of fresh fruit to hand (not cakes or biscuits).

- Each day place the money saved to one side and put it into a savings account. After 1 week you will have saved over £30, by 1 month over £120, and by 6 months at least £720, which you can spend on a well-earned holiday. Put another way, if you place the price of a packet of cigarettes at around £4 per day into an individual savings account (ISA), after 20 years the fund could be worth £44 100 (at 6% interest). In a pension plan, it could give you £4,350 (at 7% interest) per year in extra annual income! The more the price rises, the move you will save. Of course, if you carry on smoking, you may never reach your pensionable age.

- Be disciplined and don't talk yourself into smoking 'to calm me down'. If the craving is unbearable, go for a brisk walk, relax with a hot bath and drink plenty of water.

- Think positively.

- Don't carry matches or a lighter.

- Go to the dentist and have your teeth cleaned to get rid of the tobacco stains.

- Keep being positive, keep reading your reasons for quitting, reward yourself with a treat after your first week of not smoking – you've saved enough money, so go ahead!

- Avoid certain activities that are linked with smoking:

- Try to avoid alcohol and take a drink that is not associated with smoking, such as a tomato juice.

- After a meal, instead of a cigarette, clean the table, wash up, brush your teeth and go for a walk.

- Do not have cigarettes in the car; have chewing gum to hand instead.

- Outside the UK and Ireland, avoid smoky restaurants and bars.

- Holiday in countries where smoking is not allowed in public places, such as the UK or France.

- Tell your smoking friends that you will be unavailable other than on the 'phone, unless they are giving up as well.

- Keep your hands busy (fiddle with paper clips, write a letter, do the crossword, clean the car, help in the garden or with the housework).

- Use sugarless chewing gum to replace the urge to put a cigarette in your mouth.

- Take deep breaths, relax your muscles, and think of anything but cigarettes, for example your holiday plans or a previous happy experience.

- Remove everything from the house that reminds you of cigarettes: get rid of your ashtrays and matches, then have a spring clean to remove all the smell and stains of smoking, open the windows and let the fresh air circulate.

If you tell yourself you don't want to smoke rather than wishing you could smoke, you can reinforce this by noticing that your breath is better, your clothes are cleaner, the car smells better, food tastes again and that early morning cough has improved or stopped! Remember the 10 million people who have already broken the habit. The first few days are always the worst, so it does get easier! Remember that you will save over £1,825 a year.

I've given up smoking but I am afraid that I might begin again. Will it put me back to square one if I start again?

Try to avoid the urge but, if you do slip, don't despair: you can get back the ground you've lost, but you must act quickly. It is not a crime, you are not a failure, and you must not feel guilty. Look for the reason: were you tense or stressed? Were you upset or angry? Were you in a situation that you automatically associated with smoking? Then take action to avoid it happening again.

I have heard that meditation can help people to stop smoking. Do you think it works and is it worth the effort?

A lot of people benefit from learning to relax and meditate. It is particularly useful in times of stress. Relaxation tapes are available and can be helpful, as can relaxing music.

A friend of mine went to an acupuncturist to help her stop smoking and she has not smoked now for some months. I have also read that hypnosis can help. Do you think that any of these methods is any good?

There is no trial (research) evidence that acupuncture or hypnosis is effective in helping people stop smoking. However, if you are struggling, it may be worth trying either or both as they are popular with smokers and people can be helped by unproven methods. Make sure that you go to registered practitioners and keep an open mind. Always enquire about the cost before treatment begins.

I don't do much exercise. Would exercise help me to give up smoking?

Exercise is very helpful. It not only improves your overall physical condition, but it is also a great way of relieving stress and improving your mood. It takes your mind off cigarettes as well as helping to control your appetite and weight. Before you exercise, practise deep breathing and repeat this as you cool down afterwards. Dynamic exercise is best and this includes walking as briskly as possible, cycling, swimming and playing tennis or golf (see Chapter 10).

I know people who have given up smoking, but then put on weight. How can I avoid this?

People who smoke are on average 3–4 kg (7–8 lb) lighter than non-smokers. It is, however, the wrong way to stay slim. When you stop it doesn't automatically mean your weight will go up, but gaining 1 kg (2–3 lb) is not as important as quitting cigarettes.

Weight is gained when you eat more than you burn up. The trick is to watch what you eat and take up regular exercise. You need to plan positively not to let it happen.

Eat fresh fruit and vegetables; avoid cakes, chocolate and biscuits; use wholegrain cereals, porridge without sugar, pasta and bread; and drink plenty of water or low calorie drinks. You will not control your weight unless you match your intake with regular exercise – you must do both (see Chapters 9 and 10). Think of it as a lifestyle change, not a 'diet'.

It is not a good idea to stop smoking just as you go on holiday, as there will be a temptation to overeat anyway. Weigh yourself no more than once a week, at the same time of day and in the same or no clothing, to monitor your progress. Try not to become obsessed by weight. Do not start to smoke if your weight goes up; watch what you are eating and take plenty of exercise.

I've not yet tried quitting as I am frankly unable to cope with going 'cold turkey'. What can I expect as withdrawal symptoms when I stop smoking?

There is often a worsening of the smoker's cough until all the rubbish is out of your lungs. You may feel thirsty, in which case drink water and avoid caffeinated drinks and excess alcohol. Some people become constipated and hungry, and this is helped by fresh fruit and a high fibre diet (see Chapter 9). Some people become anxious, irritable and have difficulty concentrating – these feelings may last up to 4 weeks but are worse in the first 2 weeks. Drink plenty of water and take regular exercise; try to fill your time with positive activities (see the question above).

I have seen adverts for nicotine gum and patches. I smoke about 20 a day. Would nicotine replacement help me?

Some people are so addicted to nicotine that they need to be weaned off – they tend to be the people who need their first cigarette within 30 minutes of waking in the morning.

There are five sorts of nicotine replacements.

- The **patch** is like a thin plaster, which slowly gives out nicotine through the skin. It does not help if you have a sudden craving but, if you normally smoke steadily over a day, it will almost certainly suit your needs. Studies have shown that people using the patch, compared to those using a dummy patch (with no nicotine), had twice the success rate in stopping smoking. Patches come in different strengths, and heavy smokers (over 20 a day) may need to start high, weaning down to lower strengths over 2–4 weeks. Common products are Boots and Nicorette (5, 10 and 15 mg) and Nicotinell and NiQuitin CQ (7, 14 and 21 mg).

- Nicotine gum, inhalator, tablet or nasal spray help you respond to a sudden craving because they act quickly – so you may be more likely to need these if you smoke in response to sudden stress. Boots, Nicorette and Nicotinell **gum** (flavoured or plain) come in two strengths, 2 and 4 mg, and can be bought in chemist shops. Again, heavy smokers may need to start with the 4 mg strength; 8–12 pieces of either strength each day are recommended starting doses.

- The Nicorette **nasal spray** is prescription only (one spray each nostril up to twice an hour for 16 hours in every 24).

- Boots and Nicorette **inhalators** consist of a mouthpiece and replaceable nicotine cartridge – you should suck the nicotine vapour into the mouth (it does not reach the lungs). Each cartridge provides up to three 20-minute periods of intense use, and you may need 6–12 cartridges a day for 8 weeks, reducing to zero over the following 4 weeks. These can be bought in chemist shops.

- The Nicorette **tablet** (Microtab) is placed under the tongue and dissolves over 30 minutes, providing 1 mg of nicotine from a 2 mg tablet. You may need one or two every hour at first, and they can be bought in chemist shops.

The instructions must be followed carefully, and any concerns should be discussed with your family doctor or chemist. Do not use nicotine products if you are pregnant or breastfeeding.

Are there any side effects to the nicotine preparations?

For most people, side effects are not a problem. The gum may be awkward if you have dentures, and the patches may cause the skin to itch, so you may need to move them to a different place each day. The nasal spray may irritate the nose and throat and make your eyes water; the inhalator may cause a cough or irritation of the throat. The tablet can mildly irritate the mouth, but this tends to wear off with use. Sleep disturbance, vivid dreams, flushing or rashes, and nausea sometimes occur. Nicotine can upset a stomach (peptic) ulcer, so, if you are on treatment for an ulcer, check with your doctor first. If you have a history of heart attack, stroke, high blood pressure, diabetes or hardening of the arteries generally, check with your doctor first. If you are taking warfarin, inform your clinic, as there may be an interaction between the two drugs. Too much nicotine may make you feel sick, so do not smoke at the same time as using gum or patches.

Whilst combining nicotine preparations is not recommended by the manufacturers, some studies have shown improved success rates when the gum and patches, or the nasal spray and patches, are combined. Only do this after getting your doctor's advice.

Can I become addicted to the nicotine patches?

This is not a problem with the patches. However, the gum, spray, tablet or inhalator, which deal with cravings, may need to be used for over a year. When you are trying to stop using nicotine replacements, wean off gently to avoid a withdrawal reaction. You will be more successful if you combine nicotine replacement with the support of smokers' clinics and family, rather than going it alone.

How much do these products cost?

These are the approximate costs for 3 months, if you are paying yourself.

- Boots 2 mg gum £120
- Nicorette inhalator £300
- Nicorette spray £110
- Nicorette patches up to £150.

You will save your money and your life for many years ahead – think of this cost as a down payment towards better health. The good news is that nicotine replacement therapy is **now approved by the National Health Service** and is regarded as the drug treatment of choice. The family doctor and the patient must follow an agreed protocol and set a target stop date before a prescription is allowed.

I have been trying to find a support group – can they help me?

They certainly help. You will feel less alone, get support and help from others and be amongst people all trying to succeed. Phone QUIT on 020 7388 5775, or check with your local health authority for locations. QUITLINE (0800 00 22 00) provides trained counsellors to give advice, support and encouragement. The website is www.quit.org.uk (see Appendix 2).

There are now NHS helplines in England and Wales (0800 169 0169), Scotland (0800 84 84 84) and Northern Ireland (0800 85 85 85). Also try www.sickofsmoking.com to see what other smokers say. Other good sites are www.ash.org.uk and www.givingupsmoking.co.uk.

Are herbal cigarettes or dummy cigarettes worth trying?

Dummy cigarettes, such as Crave Away, Flowers or Everlasting Cigarettes, are neither harmful nor proven to be effective. Herbal cigarettes do not contain nicotine but still expose your body to tar and carbon monoxide, and are of no proven value.

Would it be better if I used a filter?

Filters can be a good idea, but unfortunately do not work for most people. Nicobrevin may help in the first weeks but should not be relied on as a long-term prop. It should be avoided if you are pregnant. Note that filters remove some of the tar but little of the risk of heart disease!

Why do some people smoke like chimneys but live a long life all the same?

Most people know someone like this. It is all about statistics: if 90% of people die from smoking, then 10% won't. The point is that the odds are against you, and trying to get away with it, or believing it can't happen to you, is courting disaster.

If someone introduced a product onto the market now that was addictive, removed oxygen from your blood, caused blood clotting, heart attacks and lung cancer, do you think they would get a licence?

I have heard a lot about Zyban. Does it help stop smoking and how does it work?

Zyban is the trade name for the drug buproprion. It is a drug used to treat depression but it was also found to help people stop smoking. How it does this is unclear but it seems to reduce the urge for nicotine and is effective for some people. It should be started 1–2 weeks before the target stop date and continued for 7–9 weeks after. It should not be used in anyone with a history of seizures (fits) or eating disorders. It also has the potential to react with some drugs. Zyban should only be used after careful discussion with your family doctor – it is available on NHS prescription.

One of my friends is taking Champix – does it work?

Champix is one of the trade names for varenicline, a new prescription-only drug which acts like nicotine and so reduces the craving for smoking. It has been shown to be very effective. You need to start it 1–2 weeks before the target stop date you agree with your doctor. The course of the treatment is about 3 months and can be repeated to prevent a relapse, though the evidence to support this is limited. Side effects include stomach upsets, dry mouth, taste disturbance, headaches, sleep disturbance, dizziness and abnormal dreams. If stopped suddenly, irritability and depression can occur. There are reports of hallucinations, suicidal thoughts and reports of suicide after starting varenicline. No definite connection with Champix has been made, but any change in mood or behaviour should be reported to your doctor.

I had a heart attack a year ago when I was 61. Is it too late to stop smoking?

It is never too late. Stopping smoking after a heart attack reduces by half your chance of having another one in the next 5 years. Stopping smoking after a heart bypass operation reduces your chances of a bypass failure over the next 10–15 years and helps prevent further disease developing.

What is a smoking cessation clinic – is it worth a try?

Special clinics and specially trained nurses and smoking cessation advisors provide support and achieve high success rates in smoking cessation (quitting). Support is usually given in groups over 6 weeks and most services also offer one-to-one counselling. Clinics take direct referrals from those wanting to stop (in a walk-in service) as well as working in partnership with family doctors. They are recommended for heavily dependent smokers needing intensive support or pregnant women especially. However, they are available to all, either in a clinic setting or as part of a local primary care service. Stopping smoking is so important: if you are having any difficulty, certainly give them a try.

RISKS OF HIGH BLOOD PRESSURE

Facts and figures

Can you tell me more about blood pressure? Why is it serious if it becomes high?

We need a blood pressure to send blood around our bodies (see Chapter 1). It is needed to overcome the resistance of the smaller blood vessels. The arteries in the body have muscle in their walls to give them tone. If this muscle is supple, the arteries can relax, their size or width increases and blood flows more easily. Think of the artery like a garden hose pipe: if you turn the tap on, water flows easily – now clamp the pipe to reduce its size by half and water will need more pressure to get through to give the same flow. In a similar way, the heart pumps the blood through the arteries but, if your arteries get smaller, the pressure will need to rise in order to force the blood through (see Figure 2.3). The top pressure, known as the *systolic pressure* (pronounced 'sis-tol-ick'), is the pressure created by your heart beating and coincides with your pulse; the bottom pressure, known as the *diastolic pressure* (pronounced 'die-a-stol-ick'), is the reading when your heart is relaxing. The readings should not be more than 140/90 mmHg. Hg is the symbol for mercury which used to be in the column of the blood pressure machine.

Blood pressure can clearly be raised at rest, for example 220/120 mmHg (when it is known as *hypertension*, see below) or normal, e.g. 120/80 mmHg, but there are areas where it is borderline, and you need regular checks to keep an eye on it. A pressure consistently above 140/90 mmHg should be investigated, but age should be taken into account as well. At 80 years this figure might be okay, but at 30 years it would not be. So although doctors talk generally of blood pressure, any decision to investigate or treat will be made on a very individual basis.

Hypertension (pronounced 'hi-per-ten-shun') is the medical word for a high blood pressure. 'Hyper' means too much, and 'tension' refers to the pressure. You may be asked to attend a hypertension clinic or a screening clinic to keep a check on your blood pressure.

What causes high blood pressure?

In the vast majority of cases there is no single cause, just as there is no single cause for people being short or tall. The medical name is *essential* or *primary hypertension*. Tests may be done to check the kidneys, adrenal gland and heart. Some people's blood pressure is raised as a side effect of their medication, particularly anti-arthritis

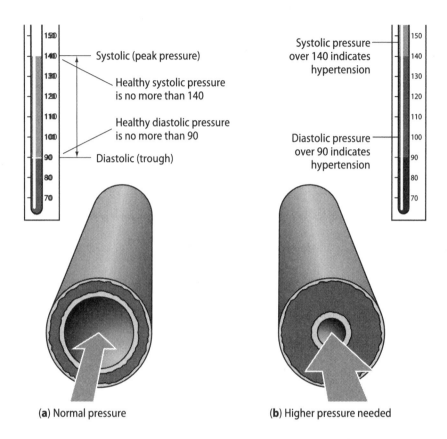

Systolic (peak pressure)

Healthy systolic pressure
is no more than 140

Healthy diastolic pressure
is no more than 90

Diastolic (trough)

Systolic pressure
over 140 indicates
hypertension

Diastolic pressure
over 90 indicates
hypertension

(a) Normal pressure

(b) Higher pressure needed

Figure 2.3 (**a**) Healthy arteries are elastic and blood flows easily
without meeting a resistance. (**b**) Arteries can lose their elasticity for
unknown reasons or suffer from disease or hardening with age.
They then become less able to relax and a higher pressure is needed
to force the blood through.

medications. Always tell your doctor or practice nurse what medicines
you have (including complementary or herbal medicines) or,
preferably, bring along any that you are taking to show your doctor.

You may have been told that you have *secondary hypertension* – this is the term used when a cause for your high blood pressure has been found (this happens in only 5% of cases). The normal or target pressure is 140/90 mmHg or less. In people with diabetes, chronic renal disease or coronary disease the target is 130/80 mmHg.

What tests can I expect to have if my blood pressure is found to be raised?

The heart may be checked with an ECG (see under *Tests* in Chapter 3) or echocardiogram (see under *Tests* in Chapter 5). A chest X-ray may be taken to look at the heart and lungs. Blood and water (urine) tests will look for any signs of anaemia (low blood count) or kidney problems, and your urine may be collected for 24 hours to see if there is too much adrenaline coming from your adrenal gland. Sometimes a scan or X-ray is taken of the kidneys.

I am not too sure what the adrenal glands are for. Can you explain their purpose?

The adrenal glands sit on top of your kidneys. They produce adrenaline. This is a hormone which speeds up your heart when you exert yourself or are emotionally excited or very frightened (white with fear), and you feel your heart pounding. Adrenaline keeps your blood pressure up if you are shocked or losing blood. Too much adrenaline that is not needed, for example in a person who is not exercising, will keep the blood pressure high unnecessarily. A tumour of the adrenal gland can do this and, although they are very rare, we check the blood or urine for excess adrenaline in younger people. If an excess is found and a tumour shown on a scan, it can be removed surgically.

My wife and I went to the doctor's to get our blood pressures checked. Hers was different to mine. Why?

Blood pressure varies from person to person and also changes in the same person. Blood pressure constantly changes within a normal range depending on what you are doing. During physical work your muscles need a greater supply of food and, to meet this extra demand, your blood flow has to be increased. To achieve this, your heart must beat faster and your blood pressure rises.

Blood pressure is lowest at night when you are asleep, but even then there are fluctuations which are presumably due to the influence of dreams. During the day the fluctuations are greater and more frequent and reflect the sort of work you are doing. Mental as well as physical stress can increase your blood pressure.

From this you will see that a doctor may need to take several readings of your blood pressure to make sure that a diagnosis of high blood pressure is a true reflection, and not due to an isolated event that could be responsible for a temporary rise in pressure. For this reason your doctor may ask you to call back to the surgery over a period of a few days or weeks in order to eliminate any temporary cause for the high level.

You can help your doctor in this respect by arriving early for your appointment, so as to avoid a rush, or worrying that you will be late. When you arrive in the surgery, relax as much as possible, because it is important to your doctor, when he is judging the level of blood pressure, to know that you are rested and calm at the time the measurement is taken (see next question).

When I went to the clinic to have my blood pressure checked, I was told that I had white coat hypertension. What is this?

This is a high reading caused by anxiety or stress when you visit your doctor –who may be wearing a white coat! At other times your blood pressure is usually normal. It may be worth checking the readings at home and during the day with a blood pressure machine that can be worn while you are walking about (an ambulatory machine; see the question later on about this.) Do several readings with your own or a borrowed machine. Blood pressure often rises under stress; throughout the day we are exposed to many stresses, so if several elevated readings occur because of environmental stress, treatment will be of value. If no elevated readings occur, your doctor should monitor your pressure regularly anyway, because we don't know if white coat hypertension is a warning for true hypertension in the future. You cannot afford to be complacent.

When I was 16, my blood pressure was lower than it is now that I am 45. Is this OK?

Yes, as a natural part of growing old, your arteries tend to lose their elastic properties to some degree. Also, the walls of your arteries tend to thicken after middle age and, consequently, the internal diameter of the vessel is slightly reduced (the hose pipe gets narrower). All these changes require a very slight increase in blood pressure, which is perfectly normal as you get older.

What are the dangers if I can't get my high blood pressure down?

If a raised blood pressure is left untreated over a 12-year period, you are more likely to die from this risk than if you had been treated. Here are some other statistics about raised blood pressure.

- It is present in 70% of people who have a stroke.
- It increases the risk of coronary heart disease by 2–3 times for men and women.
- It causes heart and kidney failure.
- It causes hardening of the arteries to the legs resulting in pain on walking owing to poor blood flow. The medical term for this is *claudication*, pronounced 'claw-dee-ca-shun'.
- It is responsible for a third of all heart diseases.

- It causes 7 out of 10 strokes in women and 4 out of 10 in men.
- In the UK, 300 people die every 6 weeks as a result of a high blood pressure and most of these deaths are avoidable; if a jumbo jet with 300 people on board crashed every 6 weeks, something would be done about it!

Are there any specific risk factors for high blood pressure that might apply to me?

You are more likely to have a high blood pressure if you:

- have someone in your family who has had high blood pressure;
- are African-Caribbean;
- are aged over 60 years of age;
- are very overweight;
- drink heavily;
- eat a lot of salt;
- had a high blood pressure in pregnancy, or pre-eclampsia;
- have a lot of stress in your life.

I have read about the rule of halves, but did not understand it. Could you explain?

This is a medical paradox but in reality it demonstrates some alarming facts about blood pressure and lack of treatment.

- Half the people with high BP have not been diagnosed.
- Half of those diagnosed have not been treated.
- Half of those treated have not got their blood pressure under control.

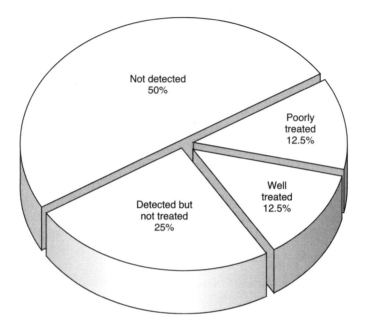

Figure 2.4 The rule of halves in people with high blood pressure: they remain poorly detected and poorly treated. Half the people with a high blood pressure do not know that they have it (not detected); half who have it may not have been told or may not have attended for treatment; half of those on treatment are not well controlled and finally half of those on treatment are properly treated and have normal pressures as a result – not a good record!

- Half of those treated are well treated.

- Only one-eighth of people with high blood pressure are being properly treated (see Figure 2.4).

So the responsibility is yours to keep nagging your doctor or practice nurse to check your blood pressure, whenever you go to the surgery. You must take charge of your own health.

How would I know if my blood pressure was raised?

Most people feel nothing until there is a problem, which is why it is known as 'the silent enemy'. It is thought that half the people with high blood pressure do not know they have it, because they cannot feel it and a doctor has not checked it. It is therefore important to have a blood pressure check every few years if it is normal, or more frequently if it is slightly raised or 'borderline'. If you go to your doctor for another reason, ask for it to be checked then.

Measurement of blood pressure

I have often seen home blood pressure monitoring machines in high street chemists, but they are pricey. Are they any good?

Some are, but others are not accurate or reliable. Ask your doctor for advice on which one to buy and then get it checked against the doctor's machine. Ask the nurse if you are not sure how to use it – go through a practice run in the surgery. Some doctors can loan you a machine for a couple of days. This is the best option because the most reliable electronic machines are the most expensive – a medical centre can buy one or two and keep an eye on their accuracy by regular checks, making sure the cuff is the right size and the batteries fresh. Digital monitors have a cuff, which inflates and deflates at the touch of a button. The Omron has been approved and validated but, for up-to-date advice, contact the British Hypertension Society (see Appendix 2).

How is blood pressure measured in the clinic?

Your doctor or nurse takes the blood pressure with an instrument called a *sphygmomanometer* (often abbreviated to *sphyg*). It is pronounced 's-fig-mo-man-omeater'. The Greek word for pulse is *sphygmos* and it is the appearance and disappearance of the pulse at the elbow that the doctor or nurse listens for (see Figure 2.5).

While your arm is relaxed and resting on a desk or supported by the doctor or nurse, a rubber cuff is wound round your upper arm just above the elbow. If your arm is large, a big cuff will be used. The cuff is attached to a column of mercury. The cuff is inflated by air being pumped into the cuff; you will feel a squeezing. The pressure in the cuff is increased until the blood flow to your hand is cut off (you may feel a tingling or numbness). Whilst the doctor listens with a stethoscope to the artery at the elbow (the *brachial artery*, pronounced 'brake-e-al'), the pressure in the cuff is lowered. The level of mercury shown in the column when the blood begins to flow again (felt as a thumping) is measured as the *systolic pressure* and, when no noises are heard (you don't feel this), it is measured as the *diastolic pressure*. Always ask what your reading is and keep your own records.

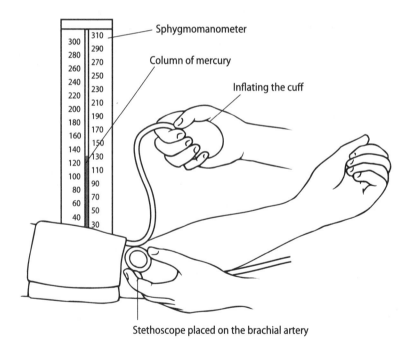

Figure 2.5 Getting your blood pressure checked in the surgery.

The mercury sphyg is being replaced by electronic measuring devices. Your practice may have changed to automatic machines but the cuff will still be put on your arm above the elbow; the wrist devices are not accurate.

How often should my blood pressure be checked?

Once a year if it is normal – try and make a note in your diary to make an appointment for the following year. If it is raised, your doctor will take several readings and keep an eye on it until it is normal. Your blood pressure will then be checked at regular intervals, usually every 3–6 months. Make sure that you ask for this measurement at least twice a year.

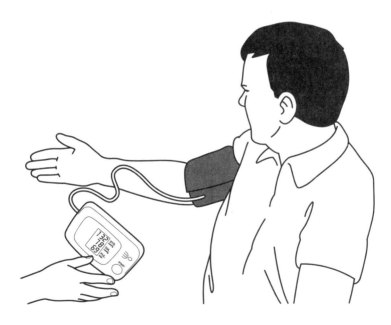

Figure 2.6 An electronic measuring device for blood pressure.

My doctor tells me that my systolic pressure is very high, although the diastolic pressure is normal. Does this matter?

It used to be thought that only the diastolic blood pressure rise was important, but modern research has shown that in people over the age of 45 years, the rise in systolic blood pressure over the normal of 140, and certainly over 160, is an important cause of subsequent heart disease and strokes. Treatment of this rise in systolic blood pressure is an important factor in reducing the risk of these serious complications.

Self-help

My mother had high blood pressure and she suffered a stroke when she was 65. Can I avoid having hypertension myself?

First of all, if someone in your family has had high blood pressure, make sure that you and your relatives have regular check-ups. Although you may feel no benefit now, you may help to prevent illness in the future, so adopt a positive approach: for yourself and those you care about. Other ways of helping yourself include:

- a healthy diet (see Chapter 9);
- exercise (see Chapter 10);
- avoiding getting overweight;
- avoiding excess alcohol;
- avoiding eating excess salt.

I'm 62 and my doctor is making me cut down on salt as she says that I am getting more sensitive to salt. What does this mean?

People over 60 years, African-Caribbeans and American Blacks have been found to have less tolerance to too much salt.

Salt-sensitive people can lower their systolic and diastolic blood pressure by 5–10 mmHg by cutting down on salt. Most, however, get a benefit of up to 4 mmHg, but every little bit helps to lower blood pressure and reduce the need for medication.

My husband has been told that he has a high blood pressure. The doctor gave him a diet sheet. How can a better diet help him?

Your husband should not overeat as, apart from anything else, this will make him put on weight, and being overweight is a major risk factor for and cause of high blood pressure. The single most important thing anybody with high blood pressure can do to help themselves is to lose weight. In some lucky people the raised pressure disappears completely and, in others, fewer tablets may be needed. If your husband is overweight, a reducing diet to get him to an optimum weight is an essential part of treatment. Losing 1 kg in weight could take 2 mmHg off his systolic blood pressure reading, so losing 3 kg (half a stone) can make a borderline pressure normal. However, his pressure will still need watching and will go back up again if the weight is put back on. See Chapter 9 for advice on a healthy diet and how to lose weight.

Treatment

I am bitterly disappointed because I have lost weight and reduced my salt intake, but I have been told that my blood pressure is still raised. What should I do?

You will need medication. Lowering your blood pressure to normal removes your chances of having a stroke and protects your heart, brain and kidneys from damage.

The good news is that treatment is very effective. Controlling high blood pressure helps prevent all the problems developing and restores you to a normal life expectancy. We now have many effective medications available to treat hypertension that need to be taken only

Table 2.2 Common drugs for raised blood pressure

Generic (real) name	Trade name (can vary in different countries)
Diuretics	
bendroflumethiazide (bendrofluazide)	Aprinox, Neo-NaClex
chlortalidone (chlorthalidone)	Hygroton
hydrochlorothiazide	Hydrenox, Hydrosaluric
indapamide	Natrilix
Potassium-sparing diuretics	
amiloride	Usually in combination
triamterine	Dytac
spironolactone	Aldactone
Beta-blockers	
acebutolol	Sectral
atenolol	Tenormin
bisoprolol	Emcor, Cardicor
carvedilol	Eucardic
celiprolol	Celectol
labetalol	Trandate
metoprolol	Betaloc, Lopresor
nebivolol	Nebilet
pindolol	Visken
propranolol	Beta-Prograne, Inderal
timolol	Betim
Calcium antagonists	
amlodipine	Istin
diltiazem	Tildiem, Adizem, Dilzem
felodipine	Plendil
isradipine	Prescal
lacidipine	Motens
lercanidipine	Zanidip
nicardipine	Cardene SR
nifedipine	Adalat, Adalat LA, Cardilate MR, Coracten XL,
nisoldipine	Syscor MR
verapamil	Securon, Cordilox, Univer

Generic (real) name	Trade name (can vary in different countries)
ACE inhibitors	
captopril	Capoten, Acepril
cilazapril	Vascace
enalapril	Innovace
fosinopril	Staril
lisinopril	Carace, Zestril
moexipril	Perdix
perindopril	Coversyl
quinapril	Accupro
ramipril	Tritace
trandolapril	Gopten
Alpha-blockers	
doxazosin	Cardura
indoramin	Baratol
prazosin	Hypovase
terazosin	Hytrin
Angiotensin II antagonists	
candesartan	Amias
irbesartan	Aprovel
losartan	Cozaar
olmesartan	Olmetec
telmisartan	Micardis
valsartan	Diovan
Combination products	
atenolol + chlorthalidone	Tenoret 50, Tenoretic
atenolol + nifedipine	Tenif, Beta-Adalat
captopril + hydrochlorothiazide	Capozide, Acezide
enalapril + hydrochlorothiazide	Innozide
lisinopril + hydrochlorothiazide	Zestoretic
losartan + hydrochlorothiazide	Cozaar-Comp
metoprolol + hydrochlorothiazide	Co-Betaloc
propranolol + bendrofluazide	Inderetic
perindopril + indapamide	Coversyl Plus
irbesartan + hydrochlorothiazide	Co Aprovel
valsartan + amlodipine	Exforge

Table 2.3 Blood pressure-lowering drugs and their possible side effects

Drug type	Possible side effects
Beta-blockers	Cold hands and feet with or without numb feeling (pins and needles); lethargy, poor concentration; heavy legs (like a zombie); wheezing; dry eyes; vivid dreams
Diuretics	Impotence; rashes; gout; possible problems for people with diabetes; muscle cramps; spironolactone: swollen or painful breasts
Calcium antagonists	Flushing, headaches and dizziness; swollen ankles which may be painful; bloated feeling and constipation
ACE inhibitors	Dry hacking cough; rash; stomach upsets
Alpha-blockers	Tiredness; dizziness; dry mouth
Angiotensin II antagonists	No major or common ones reported
Drugs that act on the brain (e.g. methyldopa, moxonidine)	Weakness, drowsiness, dizziness on standing; dry mouth; depression; impotence

once a day; if one causes a side effect, there is no need to despair because we have lots of choices and we can always find another drug that lowers the pressure to suit you.

There seem to be a lot of different medications on the market for raised blood pressure. Why have I been given one and not another?

There are various types of medications in common use. Table 2.2 lists the most commonly prescribed medications for raised blood pressure and Table 2.3 lists some of their possible side effects. The drugs have a generic or chemical name and a trade name under which they may be marketed. The trade names vary between countries so always check against the generic name to make sure that you are on the recommended medication.

Diuretics or 'water tablets' are commonly used. They remove excess salt and water from the body. They can also wash out too much potassium (and this may cause cramps) which can be dangerous if digoxin is also being taken. In some people, diuretics cause gout, and if you have diabetes they can raise your blood sugar, upsetting control of your diabetes. Common medications in this group include bendroflumethiazide, indapamide (Natrilix) and chlortalidone (Hygroton) To reduce the loss of potassium, so-called potassium-sparing agents can be prescribed and these include spironolactone, triamterene or amiloride. These two sorts of medications may be combined, as in Aldactide, Moduretic or Dyazide, in order to try and get the best results. Diuretics in general are safe and effective and side effects are not common. Fresh fruit is a good way of replacing potassium – a banana a day may do the trick.

Beta-blockers are now less frequently prescribed. These act to slow your heart rate and lower your blood pressure by blocking the effects of adrenaline. Commonly used medications are atenolol (Tenormin), metoprolol (Betaloc, Lopresor) and bisoprolol (Cardicor). The commonest side effects are cold hands and feet, heavy legs, lethargy and a 'zombie-like' feeling. Beta-blockers may cause wheezing and are not used in people with asthma. They may also hide the signs of a low sugar level in people with Type 1 (insulin-dependent) diabetes. They do not tend to mask the perspiration that goes with a hypoglycaemic attack (low sugar episode), so this warning sign is preserved. If the diabetes is stable and well controlled, they are used, but more often if there is also angina present (see Chapter 3).

As a group, the beta-blockers are useful medications, and although they are no longer first line, if you have had a heart attack you may live longer if you are prescribed them. They can be combined with diuretics for an additive effect and may be available with a diuretic in a single tablet, such as Tenoretic.

Calcium antagonists act to expand the arteries, making it easier for blood to flow (like widening the hose pipe). They can be used with diuretics and some can be used with beta-blockers. The exception is verapamil (Securon, Cordilox, Univer) as the heart rate can get dangerously slow. Calcium antagonists are helpful if you have asthma, and do not affect the medications that you may be receiving if you have diabetes. Commonly prescribed medications are amlodipine (Istin), diltiazem (Tildiem, Adizem, Dilzem), nifedipine (Adalat), verapamil (Securon) and felodipine (Plendil). Side effects include water retention (causing swollen ankles and legs), headaches, constipation (especially verapamil), occasional palpitations and sore gums. Impotence is unusual. Again these are useful medications which seem to be of more value in the elderly and African-Caribbeans. Older people and African-Caribbeans have a different hormone pattern from the kidneys, which makes calcium antagonists more effective.

ACE inhibitors and angiotensin II (AII) antagonists are widely used. ACE stands for angiotensin-converting enzyme. This enzyme is normally present in the body; blocking it causes the blood vessels to relax (the blood pressure falls as it meets less resistance) and reduces salt and water retention. Angiotensin II antagonists act in the same way but at a different point from ACE inhibitors – the end result is the same but the cough side effect of the ACE inhibitors (see below) is usually avoided.

ACE inhibitors include captopril (Capoten, Acepril), lisinopril (Carace, Zestril) and enalapril (Innovace), whilst the AIIs include

CORONARY HEART DISEASE | 47

losartan (Cozaar) and valsartan (Diovan). They both act much the same way by blocking chemicals that constrict the arteries and retain salt and water. If you have heart failure, ACE inhibitors and AIIs can lengthen your life and can protect people with diabetes from kidney damage. The main side effect is a dry hacking cough. These are important medications which have few side effects and are not known to interfere with your quality of life. AIIs do not usually cause problems with men's erections. ACE inhibitors have recently been shown to benefit patients with coronary artery disease in the absence of high blood pressure or heart failure.

Alpha-blockers act on nerve receptors to dilate the arteries – this in turn lowers the blood pressure. Prazosin (Hypovase) and doxazosin (Cardura) are the most common ones. They can cause tiredness and dizzy feelings. Their major advantage is the reduction in prostate symptoms in a man. They can be combined with all the other medications and are safe in people with asthma or diabetes.

Renin inhibitors are a new class of drugs that inhibit renin, a kidney hormone. Aliskiren (Rasilez) is now available and acts like ACE inhibitors and AIIs, relaxing the arteries. Diarrhoea can occur and checks on kidney function and blood tests for potassium are advised. Its role at present is limited.

I read in the newspaper and saw a report on TV that calcium antagonists can be dangerous – is this true?

Unfortunately for reasons that are not clear, there were scare stories about calcium antagonists. The evidence has been refuted by other researchers who looked at the claims in depth. Very high doses of nifedipine capsules can cause angina because of the speed of action of this preparation, but the capsules are not used routinely and very rarely in high doses. Claims made of an increased risk of heart attack or cancer do not stand up to careful scientific scrutiny –the claims are so devoid of scientific fact that the stories should not have been put out publicly. Much of what has been written about the dangers of calcium antagonists is nonsense and this has upset many patients and doctors. There is no danger if you take long-acting calcium antagonists, e.g. amlodipine, nifedipine LA (long-acting), and diltiazem LA, but you should avoid short-acting formulations, e.g. nifedipine capsules. The calcium antagonist scares are a classical example of media hype with commercial undertones.

Someone told me that one particular medication for blood pressure makes your hair grow – is this true?

Yes. Minoxidil is a very potent treatment used only in severe resistant blood pressure cases. It can make people put on weight because of water retention and is not used routinely for this reason. It also makes your hair grow – this can be an advantage in bald men but is not usually liked by women!

You have not mentioned Aldomet. I am pregnant and my doctor prescribed this medication for my blood pressure. Why did she choose this rather than the others that you have talked about?

Methyldopa (Aldomet) is an old and effective drug for lowering blood pressure but it does have a large number of side effects. It can cause drowsiness, sluggishness, a dry mouth, depression and impotence (see Chapter 8). Because of these effects, it is not used so much these days and has been replaced by more user-friendly medications. However, it is effective and its main use today is for raised blood pressure in pregnancy, as the medication does not cause harm to your baby. It is usually stopped on delivery to reduce the chances of depression following the birth.

I've read about a new medication called Physiotens which was called a breakthrough for blood pressure treatment in my newspaper. Should I get my doctor to put me on it?

Physiotens is the trade name for moxonidine. It acts via the brain and is advised for mild to moderate hypertension if other drugs are not appropriate or are not fully effective. Side effects include dry mouth, headache, fatigue, dizziness and sleep disturbance. It has an effective but limited place in treatment.

When I went to see my doctor, he measured my blood pressure and put me on tablets straight away. Why was this?

If your blood pressure was very high when it was first measured, it would be unlikely that changing your lifestyle alone would help. However, it is worth trying the measures discussed in the section *Self-help* earlier because these may help to reduce the amount of tablets you need.

I have been feeling tired and lethargic lately. Do you think my tablets are causing the problem?

All medications can cause side effects. We try hard as doctors to prescribe the safest and most convenient medications. If you are concerned that a particular medication is causing a problem, let your doctor know. It may have occurred by chance but it may also be associated with your treatment and a change in your medicine could relieve the symptoms. For instance, if you feel that your sex life has been affected, it may be due to your medications.

I am on treatment for high blood pressure. I know that some medications cause side effects. What should I look for?

If you feel unwell and are taking tablets, do not stop or modify your treatment in any way, but contact your doctor. He will advise what changes or modifications are necessary. This is an important point to remember because a sudden stoppage of treatment can produce what is called a 'rebound effect' in the level of blood pressure (it shoots up).

Seek your doctor's advice if you experience any of the following symptoms, but do not alter your treatment on your own.

- headaches

- visual disturbances (blurred vision)

- shortness of breath

- chest pain

- altered ability to concentrate

- memory loss

- passing more urine at night

- sexual problems/erectile dysfunction (impotence)

Remember that some of these symptoms are just as likely to be due to your blood pressure rising as to it being overtreated, so you may need to change, reduce or increase your tablets.

I have heard that blood pressure pills can affect your sex life – is this true?

The short answer is sometimes. The usual complaint is of men failing to get an erection firm enough or lasting long enough for sexual intercourse. Blood pressure itself can cause this problem and only occasionally are the drugs used to treat it, e.g. diuretics, incriminated. If it is drug-induced it will occur in the first 2–4 weeks of therapy and a different drug can then be tried. The least likely drugs to cause male erectile dysfunction (ED) are the AII antagonists (see Table 2.2) and the alpha-blockers. Female problems with lack of arousal have been reported with beta-blockers. Both men and women can get sexual problems as a result of heart disease and sometimes its treatment; if you have a problem, talk about it with your doctor or practice nurse. There is more on this subject in Chapter 8.

While I am taking my tablets, can I lead a normal life or is there anything I should avoid doing?

Although treatment controls blood pressure effectively throughout the day, it is only sensible to avoid as much as possible any events or circumstances that increase your blood pressure, such as highly emotional or stressful situations (see the section *Stress* below)

Keep your weight under control (Chapter 9), moderate your alcohol, fat and salt intake and give up cigarettes if you smoke; you should then be able to live as normal a life as possible, including a normal sex life. Above all, you should not consider yourself an invalid – you are not!

I am told that I have high blood pressure and need treatment, but I don't seem to have any symptoms. If I do not feel unwell, why should I need it?

Very often high blood pressure does not make you feel ill. This is possibly because the increase has been gradual over such a long time that you have adjusted to it. However, all the evidence shows that, if high blood pressure is left untreated, you have a greater chance of stroke, heart attacks and complications in the kidneys and eyes. When blood pressure is treated, there is overwhelming evidence that these risks are substantially reduced. Therefore, it is important, and in your interest, to take your medication exactly as prescribed by your doctor, even though you may feel quite well.

Now that I have been prescribed tablets, how long will my treatment last?

The treatment for high blood pressure, whether by lifestyle changes or drugs or both, continues for life, but as many of the medications used in its treatment need to be taken only once daily, interference with your normal lifestyle can be kept to a minimum in the majority of cases. Sometimes, if you have reached your target weight, you may have your tablets reduced or stopped, in order to see if you still need them. Ask your doctor if this is worth a try for you.

I don't mind taking one tablet a day, but one of my friends has so many that she rattles. Will these tablets be all that I need to take?

Most blood pressure patients end up on more than one medication. With some patients other factors or conditions may complicate the situation and treatment for these may also be required; you may then have to take several tablets a day. For example, if you develop angina, the tablets may need to be changed to relieve you of your chest pain (see the section *Treatment* in Chapter 3). If you develop diabetes, specific diabetic tablets may be needed. We try to tailor the treatment to the individual, aiming to keep your quality of life as good as possible – so if a diuretic causes gout, we can change to a beta-blocker, and so on. We try to give you the minimum of inconvenience, but also to keep you in good health.

My blood pressure seems to be resistant to many drugs and I have now been put on spironalactone. How is this different?

Spironalactone is a diuretic (water tablet) that antagonises a hormone called aldosterone. It can be very useful when the blood pressure is proving difficult to control. Kidney function needs to be monitored, and as it retains potassium caution is needed if used with ACE inhibitors or AIIs. The commonest side effects are stomach upsets and swollen breasts, mainly in men (gynaecomastia), which can be painful. Erection problems in men, and period changes in women, can also occur.

What should I do if I forget to take my tablets?

For most people, there is no need to worry, as the blood pressure will only rise slowly, so you can get back on schedule the next day. If you are on a beta-blocker and also have angina, you should take the medication immediately you realise that you have forgotten it, as a means of catching up.

RISKS OF HIGH CHOLESTEROL LEVELS

Facts and figures

There is a lot of talk these days about lipids and cholesterol and now I've seen something about triglycerides! I am rather muddled about it all. Can you tell me what all these words mean?

Cholesterol is a fatty or oily substance and is one of a group of fatty substances we call *lipids*.

Lipids are essential for the normal functioning of the body's cells. Problems develop when there is too much lipid in the blood. It then settles in the walls of the arteries. The arteries then develop the narrowings which cause heart attacks and angina by restricting the flow of blood to the heart (see the Introduction to this chapter). Doctors often ask for a 'lipid profile': this is a check on the levels of cholesterol and triglycerides in your blood. (Triglyceride is another fatty substance – see below).

Cholesterol plays an essential role in helping our glands make hormones, but its biggest role is in the formation of cell walls. We are able to make all the cholesterol we need in the liver, where it is made from fat. Our problems begin if we have a higher blood cholesterol than we need; this is usually due to eating too much fat (see the question later on *hypercholesterolaemia*).

Triglycerides (pronounced 'try-gli-sir-ides') are the major form of saturated fats (see later question) which come from food and they are also made in the body to provide energy. If you have a high level of triglycerides and a low level of high density lipoproteins (see next question), you have a greater chance of developing coronary disease. Triglycerides are commonly raised in people who are very overweight, people with diabetes and those who have a high alcohol intake.

I was told that all cholesterol is bad for you. Now I read that there is a 'good' cholesterol and 'bad' cholesterol. What's the difference?

Cholesterol and other fats do not dissolve in the blood. They hitch a ride on proteins which are the taxis transporting the fats around. The combination of fat and protein is a *lipoprotein* (pronounced 'lie-po-pro-teen'). The 'bad' cholesterol is the low density lipoprotein (LDL): this is the main carrier of harmful cholesterol to your arteries where it builds up to cause narrowings. The high density lipoproteins (HDL) are the good guys: HDL tends to pick up excess cholesterol taking it away from the arteries and transporting it back to the liver for removal. So, for maximum protection, you need:

- your LDL low (L for lousy);

- your HDL high (H for happy).

I'm going to have a complete check-up next month. When I have my cholesterol profile checked, what levels should all these different fats be?

Your total cholesterol should not be above 5.0 mmol/litre. The HDL (see question above) should be greater than 1.0 mmol/L in a man, and 1.3 mmol/L in a woman.

The LDL should be 3.0 mmol/L or less – the ideal is 2.6 or less.

Your *triglycerides* should be less than 1.7 mmol/L, ideally 1.6 or less.

As a rule of thumb, a total cholesterol of 5.0 equals an LDL of 3.0.

However, for coronary patients and those with chronic renal disease or diabetes, the targets are lower:

- cholesterol 4 mmol/L or less;

- LDL 2.0 mmol/L or less.

So remember 5 and 3, and 4 and 2.

Research has shown that lowering cholesterol to these levels in normal people, as well as in coronary patients, helps prevent heart disease in the future. The benefits apply to both men and women.

When I had a lipid profile done on my blood, the doctor told me I had hypercholesterolaemia. What does this mean?

*H*ypercholesterolaemia (pronounced 'hi-per-kol-esterol-eemia') means that the total cholesterol is high in the blood. Usually the LDL (see question above) is raised; in women the HDL is higher before the menopause – an effect of their hormones. It is always better to know both profiles (HDL and LDL), as well as the total level, because you don't want to lower a high HDL by mistake. For example, a woman before the menopause may have a high total cholesterol (e.g. 5.8) which is made up mainly of the good HDL (e.g. 2.0).

When I look at a food label, there are different types of fats listed, such as saturated and unsaturated fats. Can you explain more about the differences between the types of fats?

There are two main sorts of fats.

- *Saturated fats* are mainly of animal origin. They are the bad fats and it is the saturated fat that raises your cholesterol levels.

- *Unsaturated fats* are mainly of vegetable origin and they lower your cholesterol levels.

Saturated fats are a mixture of alcohol, glycerol and fatty acids. The fatty acids contain long chains of carbon atoms – most commonly 12, 14 or 16. These are the most effective at raising the LDL ('bad cholesterol') in the blood. The more saturated fat we eat, the higher the cholesterol; if we eat less, our cholesterol will fall over 3–4 weeks. *Unsaturated fats* contain carbon atoms that are joined (with double bonds) at certain points; this leads to the fats being liquid or soft at room temperature. When there is one double bond, the fat is *monounsaturated*; when there are two or more, it is *polyunsaturated*. Monounsaturated fats include olive, rapeseed and peanut oils and are contained in avocados, almonds and oily fish. Polyunsaturated fats include sunflower oil and most soft margarines (always read the label!). Polyunsaturated fats help prevent blood clots forming, which is another benefit in addition to their cholesterol-lowering effect.

As well as lowering your LDL (bad) cholesterol by switching you away from saturated fat, unsaturated fats also appear to have an additional good effect on lowering cholesterol. Monounsaturated fat may raise the HDL (good) cholesterol as well. All kinds of fat, whether saturated or unsaturated, are rich in calories, so you need to bear in mind, when you change to a healthy diet, not to go overboard on unsaturated fat.

Chapter 9 gives lots of information about which foods contain the different types of fats and gives you lists from which you can choose a healthy diet.

The media has also talked about the harmful effects of trans fatty acids. How can I avoid them?

Trans fatty acids are present in small quantities in meat and dairy products but are present in larger quantities in those oils which have been manufactured to be firmer at room temperature (i.e. when oils have been made into margarines or spreads) by a process known as *hydrogenation*. Trans fatty acids raise LDL and lower HDL cholesterol levels. When you are selecting vegetable oils and margarine it is important to look for the trans content. The best oils are blended vegetable oils, rapeseed oil and soft margarines that are low in saturates and trans fatty acids, but high in polyunsaturates and mono-unsaturates (see the question above). Always read the margarine label.

The article that I read also mentioned vitamin E as being beneficial. Why is it important?

V itamin E is an *antioxidant*; antioxidants help protect the body from 'free radicals'. *Free radicals* are produced by some of the normal chemical reactions in the body cells. They are unstable and, in excess, can damage the lining of the cells by oxidising LDL ('bad') cholesterol, causing it to stick to the walls of the arteries.

Antioxidants are present in fruit and vegetables and can prevent cholesterol being oxidised so that it does not tend to stick to the artery wall.

Some early studies suggested that vitamin E protects against heart disease, but unfortunately subsequent studies have not shown any benefit from tablet supplements. Vitamin E is present in food containing a lot of polyunsaturates, such as vegetable oils (especially sunflower) and deep green leafy vegetables. Nuts and vegetable oils, although good sources of vitamin E, are also high in calories, so these should not be eaten too frequently. There is a small amount of vitamin E in wholemeal bread. Some margarines are enriched with vitamin E. If your food intake is high in polyunsaturates, it will contain a lot of vitamin E. Because some of the major sources are high in calories, you may be advised to take extra vitamin E as supplementary tablets by some specialists to avoid putting on weight, but for most of us this will not be necessary. Chemists and health food shops sell vitamin E preparations and the recommended dose is 100–200 units a day (70–140 mg). However, as vitamin supplements have been shown to be of no benefit – save your money!

You have talked about vitamin E. What about vitamin C – isn't this an antioxidant as well?

Y es, and it is safe to take, but medical trials have demonstrated no benefit for heart disease. It is found in citrus fruits (oranges, grapefruits, lemons), kiwi fruit, soft fruit (strawberries, raspberries, blackberries), red and green peppers and spring greens. Try to eat

150–200 g (6–8 oz) of this group a day and you will not need tablet supplements.

I have always believed taking vitamin supplements would protect me – are you saying this is not true?

Unfortunately yes. The Heart Protection Study involved thousands of patients and those taking vitamins did no better or worse than those taking placebos (fakes). In other words, vitamins do not protect against the effects of hardening of the arteries and are of no benefit to the heart. The vitamin story is a good example of an idea that is theoretically good but, when tested, does not work.

I know of people taking beta carotene supplements and our health food shop is always marketing it. What is beta carotene, and should I be taking it?

No. Beta carotene is converted in the body to vitamin A. It is an antioxidant and is found in brightly coloured fruit and vegetables (carrots, broccoli, tomatoes, melons, yellow and orange peppers, spinach, peaches). So you might think that extra supplements would be good for you. However, medical trials have failed to show that they have any benefit, and researchers are now worried that they may lead to an increased risk of some cancers and heart disease. Do not waste your money on beta carotene supplements – fruit and vegetables are all that you need.

I thought that people supplementing their diet with extra beta carotene from the health food shops had a lower chance of developing heart disease or cancer. You say that there may be risk of developing these conditions – which view is right?

This question is a good example of the need always to make sure that a good idea works when put into practice. Beta carotene has antioxidant properties and, in theory, could help prevent cancer and coronary heart disease. Indeed, people who took beta carotene supplements were *observed* to be less likely to develop these diseases – but an observation is not proof. Four research studies involving thousands of people set out to prove whether a benefit existed when beta carotene was compared to placebo (see the section *Other treatments for angina* in Chapter 3). These were proper scientific studies. Surprisingly and alarmingly, beta carotene supplements were shown to increase heart disease and cancer risks, especially in smokers and people exposed to asbestos. Ideas, whether based on good scientific theory, as in the case of beta carotene, or dreamed up in the bath, should always be validated! Beta carotene should be consumed normally in fresh fruit and vegetables.

There is so much advice about fat intake that I really don't know what to believe. How much fat should we eat a day?

This depends on whether you need to reduce weight, that is, reduce calories. Remember that fat, whether good (unsaturated) or bad (saturated) is high in calories. We need 50–90 g of fat a day of which 22–27 g, only, should be saturates. Always look on the food labels to help you choose foods that contain less saturated fats.

Let's work out some numbers. Doctors recommend that no more than 30% of your calorie intake is fat, and 10% of that is saturated fat, regardless of whether or not you are overweight. If your daily calorie intake is 1500 kcal, this means 50 g of fat at most (1 g of fat equals 9 kcal). If your daily calorie intake is 2000 kcal, this means 65–70 g of fat; if it is 2500 kcal, this means 85–90 g of fat. (See Chapter 9 for further information on fats in food.)

My father had a high cholesterol level and died aged 55. My wife is concerned that I may be like him – I am now 52. Can this be inherited?

Some people may inherit a high cholesterol level (usually over 8.0 mmol/litre). A good diet changes these people's levels only marginally and they will need medication. Make sure that all members of your family are checked for an inherited pattern and, if this is detected, you will be recommended medication. Other people inherit a tendency to a high cholesterol level but respond to diet, plant stanols or, more usually, a combination of diet and medications.

Self-help

Should I know my cholesterol and other test level numbers? Will it do any good?

If you want to reduce your chances of heart disease, you must take charge of your lifestyle, and that includes knowing your numbers and keeping track of how they respond to any changes in your eating pattern or medication.

How well will a healthy diet lower my cholesterol?

A healthy diet may reduce your cholesterol by 10%. Obviously the higher your cholesterol at the start, the more likely you will need medications as well, but a period of healthy diet restricting your fat intake for 3 months is normally recommended first (see Chapter 9). However, if you already have heart problems, most doctors advise immediate medication to take full advantage of its cholesterol-lowering effect.

Which is more important – to avoid foods high in cholesterol or saturated fats?

Cholesterol in your food has a smaller effect on the blood cholesterol level than do foods high in saturated fat. It is more important therefore to cut down on foods high in saturated fat. This means, for example, that you can have three to four eggs a week (the yolks are high in cholesterol). Cutting down on saturated fat (and all fats) will help you to lose weight (see Chapter 9).

I am told that I have a high cholesterol level. If I manage to lower this level, will this really prevent heart disease?

We now have overwhelming evidence that lowering your cholesterol level not only reduces your risks of heart disease by an average of over 30%, but also reduces the need for heart bypass surgery and angioplasty (see Chapter 3). If you lower your cholesterol over a 5-year period, you improve your chances of living longer by an amazing 30%. Treating a high cholesterol is one of the most important means of preventing and reducing the complications of coronary artery disease. Some doctors believe it is negligent not to lower a raised cholesterol.

What should I get my cholesterol levels down to in order to see a benefit to my heart?

Most of the benefit occurs when the LDL ('bad') cholesterol is lowered by 30% or more; your aim should be to get this level below 3.0 mmol/litre with an ideal of 2.0 mmol/litre, or less if you have coronary disease, diabetes or a chronic renal condition. This leads to removal of the soft part of the narrowings in the arteries making them less likely to tear or split. It is known as stabilising the plaque (see the Introduction to this chapter). Unstable plaque that ruptures releases soft cholesterol into the blood which then causes a clot to form and a possible heart attack to occur – removing the soft cholesterol helps to prevent this happening.

I have reduced my cholesterol level so that the tests are now normal. Can I go back to smoking?

No. Risk factors, which increase your chances of developing heart problems, are independent of each other. If you have more than one risk factor, however, they don't just add up, they multiply.

Table 2.4 Cholesterol-lowering drugs

Drugs	Effects	Side effects
Statins		
Atorvastatin (Lipitor)	Lower LDL by over 20% and up to 50%	Rare stomach upsets; muscle pains; sleep disturbance
Fluvastatin (Lescol)		
Pravastatin (Lipostat)		
Simvastatin (Zocor)		
Rosuvastatin (Crestor)		
Fibrates		
Fenofibrate (Lipantil)	Raise HDL, lower triglycerides (30%)	Uncommon stomach upsets; muscle pains; rash
Ciprofibrate (Modalim)		
Bezafibrate (Bezalip)		
Gemfibrozil (Lopid)		
Resins		
Colestyramine (Questran)	Lower LDL but raise triglycerides	Constipation; bloating; gas
Absorption inhibitors		
Ezetimibe (Ezetrol)	Lowers LDL cholesterol by 20%	Stomach upsets; muscle pain; headache

I have seen cholesterol self-testing kits in the chemists. Are these any good?

Not really. They are not as accurate as we had hoped they would be.

Do I need to starve for the blood test?

A blood sample which will show the levels for total cholesterol and HDL can be taken at any time, and this will be a useful screening test. However, the LDL and triglyceride levels are influenced by diet and should be measured after at least nine hours of fasting, but you can drink water.

My doctor has only measured my total cholesterol level. Is this enough, or should I ask for all the different levels to be measured?

When your doctor is giving you a screening test, the total cholesterol level is a good guide. A total cholesterol of 5.0 or less is satisfactory and remember that 5.0 of total cholesterol is equivalent to 3.0 of 'bad' LDL. However, if your doctor is planning your treatment, a full lipid profile is needed to guide therapy properly. If you are going to be on medication for a long time, you need to be sure that you are on the right type.

When should I have a repeat cholesterol level test?

When you have been on your new healthy diet for 3 months, the doctor will ask you to come in for another test.

Treatment

What happens if my second cholesterol level test is still raised?

You will need medication. Fortunately, the medications that you might be given are safe, simple to use and very effective – usually your cholesterol levels will begin to fall within 21 days.

What medications are there to treat high cholesterol levels and are there any side effects?

The commonest medications that you may be prescribed are known as the statins (see Table 2.4). They reduce the production of cholesterol in the liver. Side effects are rare but you may get indigestion, muscle aches and pains, sleep disturbance, rarely a rash, and possibly a reduced sex drive or impotence. After you have been on one of these medications for 3–4 weeks, your doctor will want to check your cholesterol again to make sure that the dose is right and that you are not suffering from any of these side effects. Always tell your doctor if you feel that you are having side effects.

The next most common group of medications is the fibrates. These are used more when your HDL is low and your triglycerides high. Stomach upsets and skin rashes occur sometimes as side effects.

Sachets of medications known as the resins are used less these days as they can cause a lot of stomach trouble and they taste like wallpaper paste (not that I have tried it) or sand. Ezetimibe acts to prevent the absorption of cholesterol and is often used when statins are not fully effective or causing side effects. It can be used in combination with statins to provide additional cholesterol lowering (see later).

A combination of medications is occasionally used to increase their effect, when a single medication is not enough to get the levels right.

I have been prescribed cholesterol-lowering medication, although I am only 50. Will I always need medication?

Usually, yes. Occasionally, after a time when you have been losing weight and eating healthily, the medication can be stopped for a month to see what happens; usually your cholesterol goes up again, but at least you've proved that you do need medication.

If you have coronary disease, lowering your cholesterol will help reduce your chances of a heart attack or the need for heart surgery or angioplasty. Lowering your cholesterol will also help to lengthen your life. For most people, one, or occasionally, two tablets a day plus a healthy lifestyle are all that is needed. The tablets are easy to take, with few side effects. This is one occasion when 'keep on taking the tablets' is very good advice and, in terms of healthcare, very good value.

When I have finally got my cholesterol level under control, how often should I have it checked?

Every 12 months.

I have been on cholesterol-lowering medication for some time now. When I go for a check-up, my doctor checks my liver. Why?

It is in the liver that the statins, in particular, get to work, and, very rarely, cause an upset; the tablets then have to be stopped. If you are unfortunate enough to have this side effect, you will be pleased to know that the liver will get better, once the medication has been withdrawn. Statins do not cause cancer.

Can lowering cholesterol levels be harmful, as I have read that lowering cholesterol increases the chances of suffering a violent death or suicide?

There were some reports suggesting this but, by proper scientific study, they have been disproved. This is called evidence-based medicine. Lowering cholesterol reduces your chance of dying from heart disease and does *not* increase your chance of dying from anything else. There is no increased risk of cancer.

I have had a heart attack and even though my cholesterol was only 4.5 I have been put on a statin – why is this?

If you have coronary disease, the level of cholesterol at which you developed it is too high for you. Studies have shown a significant benefit in reducing heart attacks, strokes or death in those with known coronary disease or those at high risk (such as those with diabetes), who start with a cholesterol as low as 3.5 mmol/litre. Statins have other properties other than lowering cholesterol and can reduce the inflammation in the narrowing of arteries, preventing disruption. So, once the disease is known about, the treatment is more aggressive because the benefits are substantial.

> *I have read about a new cholesterol drug called Ezetrol – when is this used?*

Ezetrol is the UK trade name for ezetimibe; this is a drug that acts to prevent the absorption of cholesterol in the bowel. It is a fixed dose of 10 mg and lowers LDL cholesterol by 10–20% when acting on its own or added to statin therapy. Side effects are not common – mainly nausea and bloating and occur in only 2% of people taking it. It is used when statins are not tolerated at all or when the dose needed to achieve your target for LDL cholesterol causes side effects – it can then be added to a lower dose of statin, which is tolerated, to get an additive effect. To date there is no evidence that it reduces heart attacks, so statins are the number one choice. There has been some concern about an increased cancer risk but a detailed review of the research did not confirm this. Like all new drugs, its use will be carefully supervised.

OTHER RISK FACTORS FOR CORONARY HEART DISEASE

Being overweight – obesity

> *I don't feel overweight but the doctor says I am. Have I got more chance of developing heart disease because of this?*

Very overweight (*obese*) people do have more chance of developing heart disease and this has been mentioned earlier (see the section **Risks of high blood pressure**). Being fat increases the work the heart has to do, causes high blood pressure and leads to abnormal blood lipids (*hypercholesterolaemia*). It can also lead to you developing diabetes (see below). You should try to reduce your weight – see Chapter 9 for advice about healthy eating and losing weight. Big bellies are bad for your heart!

Stress

I have a very stressful job. Am I more likely to get heart problems?

There is no proof that stress actually causes heart disease but it can contribute to the symptoms. It is like a trigger, setting things off. Stress is a state of mind, not an illness, so it is difficult to obtain a precise measurement of it. We all feel stress but it affects us in different ways and we respond differently. Under stress people may smoke or drink more, overeat for comfort or have slightly higher blood pressures.

Stress can be fun as well as unpleasant, for example watching a close team match or taking part yourself in team games. A sudden acute stressful incident is the most dangerous (such as a near-miss on the motorway) but usually cannot be avoided. Stress interacts with your chances of developing heart disease and can make them worse.

Will I be able to recognise the symptoms of dangerous levels of stress?

Symptoms will vary but, in general, when stress is detrimental, you will become tense, nervous and often afraid; you may sleep badly, wake early and have tension pains in the muscles of the neck or back.

Is there any way I can reduce my stress levels?

Yes, there are various ways you can help yourself.

- Try to remove yourself from a stressful environment for some of the day. If work is stressful, go for a walk at lunch time. Keep physically active.

- Don't rely on caffeine or alcohol and don't smoke.

- Learn that you cannot solve all life's problems alone and that they are not all caused by you.

- Try relaxation tapes, yoga or deep breathing exercises. These work well for some people (see below).

- Spend less time with people who irritate you.

- Try to avoid rush-hour travel (leave for work earlier and walk the last mile or so).

- Talk through any problems at work or with friends (don't repress them and let them fester).

- Avoid over-commitment – be positive but don't be afraid to turn things down.

- Don't rush about; take your time, plan what you are going to do and follow it through – again be positive and don't be deflected.

- Most of all, keep life in perspective – yesterday is gone, tomorrow hasn't happened, just get on with today and enjoy it.

The most important therapy is your own. Look at what you are doing and ask what your priorities are. If you had one day left in your life, would you shout and yell in traffic, or swear at the railway guard because the train is late (again!), or would you spend time with your loved ones, telling them how much they mean to you. Take deep breaths and keep the world in proportion. If you must do something, punch a pillow but laugh at yourself as you do it!

Really stressed people usually have other psychological problems which benefit from counselling or a support group. If you are unlucky enough to have a heart attack, a 'cardiac rehabilitation programme' is invariably helpful. It provides expert help and support as well as guidance on exercise and a healthy lifestyle. It is usually run by nurses who understand your fears and worries, and can help you regain your confidence.

Diffuse your feelings by using art, music, dance and exercise as a relief valve. There are many videos, tapes and books on stress management which people have found useful. Any relaxation technique will help. Yoga is a very useful exercise and is an ideal way to wind down and relax. Take evening classes which will allow you to meet others and get away from your normal daily routine.

Above all else, remember that by bringing stress under control you will not only benefit your heart but also improve your outlook on life, allowing better and more complete relationships with loved ones, friends and colleagues at work.

Why is so much emphasis placed on stress in the media?

There is a lot of money in stress management and it is an easy diagnostic dustbin. If you have a funny illness, it's 'a virus'; if you can't explain something, it's 'stress'!

I have read about type 'A' and 'B' personalities having an effect on the heart. What is the difference between them?

Some psychiatrists divide the world into two groups, type A and type B people. Type A people are competitive, intense and driven by success. Type B are relaxed, unhurried and content with their lives and achievements. Type A personality has been linked to heart disease but several studies have failed to establish a direct connection. It may well be the consequences of a type A personality that establish a relationship with heart problems, reflecting the degree of anger and frustration that these people feel rather than their attitudes and activities alone.

Do different emotions affect the heart adversely?

Anger appears to be the most dangerous emotion, increasing heart strain by raising blood pressure and increasing heart rate. If you are angry, write a letter about the person or problem, expressing your anger, then tear it up. (Don't send it!) Yell and shout at a mirror, then laugh at yourself as you regain perspective. Learn to count to 10 slowly, while breathing deeply.

I feel that I am stressed at the end of the day. What can I do?

You are probably overdoing things and overcommitted. Look at your day: can you organise it better?

- Does anyone or any issue stress you more? If so, bring it into the open.
- Walk some of the way to work and try to get out at lunch time.
- If you feel trapped in your home all day, make the effort to go out – go window shopping, walk round a shopping mall if it is raining; walk in the park if it's fine.
- Complete the day with deep breathing exercises, have a warm soak in the bath, clean your teeth and freshen up.
- Read a book, do a crossword, work on a hobby project, or 'surf the net' and think about your priorities.
- If you have a pet, pat it or stroke it – play with the cat, or walk the dog.

Stress is usually present when emotions are bottled up and everything gets out of perspective.

Diabetes

I have had diabetes for 30 years. What is the effect of diabetes on heart disease?

People with diabetes do have more heart disease than those without. Whilst very good and strict sugar control may reduce some of the risk, this is undone by an increased number of hypoglycaemic attacks. Although you can't help having diabetes and, unfortunately, it cannot yet be cured, you can help the other factors that cause heart disease. Do not smoke, keep as fit as you can and avoid getting overweight; keep your cholesterol in check and aim for a normal blood pressure.

Many doctors routinely put people with diabetes on statins to reduce the risk no matter what their cholesterol level is.

I have diabetes and have now been told that I have insulin resistance and am at risk of heart disease – what is insulin resistance?

Normally, when you eat food, your blood sugar (glucose) levels go up; your body produces insulin as a response; insulin helps glucose to be taken up by the tissues, the glucose in your blood falls, and then your insulin level falls. It is called a negative feedback mechanism. If you are insulin-resistant the action of insulin in the tissues is less effective than it should be and glucose (sugar) is not used properly, so the sugar and insulin levels remain raised because the feedback is interrupted. Insulin in high levels can raise the blood pressure, cause salt and water retention and raise LDL ('bad') cholesterol and lower HDL ('good') cholesterol. Therefore, yes, insulin resistance can increase your risks of developing heart disease.

Being overweight, particularly abdominal obesity (a fat belly), is associated with or causes insulin resistance and Type 2 diabetes. By reducing weight, both diabetes and insulin resistance can be controlled or even overcome. It is more common among Indo-Asian people. Besides reducing your weight, you can also take medications to lower insulin resistance such as metformin or other anti-diabetic drugs.

Illegal drugs

I worry that my teenage daughter might have access to drugs. Do illegal drugs affect young people's chances of heart problems?

Cannabis (or 'pot' or marijuana) increases the heart rate and blood pressure as well as body temperature. It also contains carbon monoxide in the smoke. Although it can help some medical problems, for example, the nausea of cancer therapy, severe pain and multiple sclerosis, heart problems is not one of them and it is therefore not recommended.

Cocaine ('crack') is a powerful addictive drug which can cause blood vessels to shut down (go into spasm; see Figure 2.7). It can raise blood pressure, cause strokes and lead to severe heart disease, provoking irregular heartbeats, inflaming heart muscle and causing heart attacks. Just one 'fix' can do it – my advice is don't try it.

You may have heard that *morphine* helps the heart. It is not that simple. Children may begin with the idea of taking heroin (related to morphine) in small amounts and keeping it under control, but the addiction takes over, infection risks rise (from dirty needles or impure products), the heart valves can become severely damaged and the heart, overwhelmed by disease, gives up functioning properly. This leads to heart failure, resulting in a rapid and inevitable premature death.

If you think your child may be addicted, seek help. Help is available for recovery but an addict needs to admit to addiction, want to end it and accept help from professionals.

Ecstasy has been very much in the news. Taking even one ecstasy tablet is akin to committing suicide. It may cause a very high fever, irreversible brain damage and heart failure.

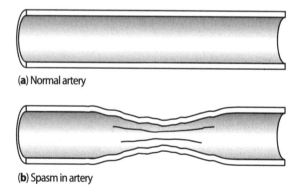

(a) Normal artery

(b) Spasm in artery

Figure 2.7 Lengthways section of (a) a normal artery and (b) an artery in spasm, which narrows the opening available for blood flow.

WOMEN AND CORONARY HEART DISEASE

I am a mother aged 53. I am concerned to read that coronary heart disease is a major risk for me. Isn't this a man's disease?

Of the deaths from heart attacks each year, nearly half are in women. All forms of heart and blood vessel diseases added together claim twice as many women's lives as do all forms of cancer. Although fewer women have heart disease than men at the age of 50, they have caught up by 65–70 years of age. The main difference between men and women as regards heart disease is not if they are going to get coronary disease, but when; the difference in its timing is about 10 years.

Coronary heart disease is therefore your – and other women's – biggest problem too. It is becoming more of a woman's disease as women tend to live longer; coronary disease is partly a problem of getting older, so more women will eventually develop it. The problem is going to increase as the population ages in general. More men and women are now surviving heart attacks, so they are likely to encounter heart problems later – an increased chance of angina or a further heart attack, unless they try to reduce their risks. Women are more vulnerable to the risks of cigarette smoking and high blood pressure but less so to that of cholesterol. Having diabetes sadly wipes out any advantages that women may have had over men (see above).

My father had heart disease and I am concerned that my daughter might develop heart disease also. I know that she smokes. How can I help her avoid heart disease?

Your daughter may have an increased risk of heart disease if it runs in your family but one of the best ways to help prevent coronary heart disease is to get her to stop smoking. It is well known that there has been an increase in the numbers of young women smoking; their chances of heart disease in later life consequently are rising. If your daughter smokes, she should stop now. If she is thinking about starting, she should think again!

I have read that women's natural hormones protect us from heart disease. Is this true?

To a degree they do, but if you smoke, have high blood pressure or have diabetes, women lose a lot of this protection. Following the menopause, the normal protection that oestrogen gives disappears anyway. Hormone replacement therapy (HRT; see below) unfortunately does not appear to help.

I have been taking the pill on and off since I was 18. I have just been through the menopause. Am I at any greater risk of heart disease because I have been using oral contraceptives?

Very few women on the pill (taking oral contraceptives) develop heart disease and the low hormone dose pills do not increase the coronary risk. So long as you do not smoke, the low dose pill may actually protect you against heart problems. In women under 35 years of age we do not know what the risk is from taking the pill, nor do we know about its long-term use (over 5 years), although it is unlikely you will be harmed. Cigarette smoking and also taking the pill is not a good combination and should be avoided at all costs. In general the low dose pills are safe, but smokers should preferably stop smoking, or use alternative contraception.

I have felt well since being on HRT but I am worried about its effect on my heart and the risk of breast cancer – what should I do?

There is no doubt that HRT helps with the distressing symptom of menopausal flushes and protects against thinning of the bones (osteoporosis). Initial enthusiasm regarding HRT and heart disease has been replaced with sound scientific evidence of a lack of benefit. Currently HRT is not recommended as a treatment to prevent heart disease developing or to benefit women who have heart disease already. If coronary disease has been diagnosed, other protective treatments should be used – for example statin therapy. Some studies have suggested HRT can actually increase the risk of heart disease, but this risk does not appear to be present if the cholesterol is normal or a statin is also being taken.

A very big study – The Million Women Study – has identified an increased risk of breast cancer if HRT is taken for 5 years or more. We are looking at 1 extra case of breast cancer in 166 women treated for 5 years or 1 extra case in 53 women treated for 10 years. There is no need to panic about these figures, but clearly women on HRT for many years should see their family doctor about discontinuing.

The HRT story is a sad journey from the belief of benefit to the proof of potential harm. There is no role for HRT in women who do not have menopausal symptoms (such as flushes). When flushes are a problem (this happens in 10–20% of women), the risks must be weighed against the benefit, and HRT used for as short a time as possible.

Most women are on combined medications of oestrogen and progestogen but, if they have had a hysterectomy (removal of the womb), they will be on oestrogen alone. All increase the breast cancer risk. With regard to the heart, we are not sure about oestrogen alone but, with all the information we have, HRT cannot be considered a treatment for heart disease.

Whether this advice will change when we know more about raloxifene (see next question) is debatable, but it is obviously important to continue research in this area and advise women on up-to-date scientific facts.

I have read in the paper about a new drug called raloxifene – what advantage does this have?

Raloxifene is one of a class of drugs called Selective Estrogen (American spelling) Receptor Modulators, or SERMS. Tamoxifen is the one we already have but tamoxifen can sometimes, as a side effect, cause the uterus (womb) lining to overgrow and become troublesome. Raloxifene acts the same as tamoxifen in benefiting the heart and bones, avoids breast cancer risks and does not affect the womb. It is an important drug but like tamoxifen does not reduce hot flushes. It may be an important advance in HRT for women because it looks to have the major benefits without the major risks. A lot of research is taking place to determine how valuable it will be to the heart – proof is not yet available, but early results do not show any harm.

Does HRT have any side effects?

All medication can give side effects and HRT is no exception. You may feel nauseous but it usually goes after 2 weeks or so – taking tablets after a meal can help this. Breast tenderness and swelling may occur and, again, wear off. If they are persistent, you may be given a different form of HRT to try.

Women worry about gaining weight whilst on HRT. The many research trials do not report weight gain but you should remember that everyone is an individual and if you gain weight, it is you that matters, not the statistics. It is probably due to eating more as you feel better on HRT! Watching your weight is important anyway, so at this time take note of what you are eating and make sure that you take plenty of exercise.

On average, women take 3 months to settle into their HRT therapy.

Does HRT raise blood pressure?

Very rarely. Your doctor or nurse will always check your blood pressure when HRT is prescribed. If you have high blood pressure, you can still take HRT because the chances of your control being upset are so small.

I have breast cancer which is now controlled, and I have also had a heart attack – will HRT help me?

It will not obviously help the heart and it could make the breast cancer worse, so it is not recommended. HRT is not an alternative to proven heart attack treatments.

What sort of HRT therapy is available?

The choice of therapy is best discussed with your doctor. There are two sorts: the first is oestrogen only and this type is for women who have had a hysterectomy (removal of the womb) – this is known as 'unopposed oestrogen'. The second type is 'combined' HRT (containing oestrogen and progesterone) for women who still have a womb, because oestrogen alone in these women will cause excess stimulation of the lining of the womb.

I have been advised to go on HRT but I am resisting as I have read that it doubles your chances of getting blood clots in the legs – is this true?

Yes, this is true. Your normal risk of getting a dangerous blood clot is 1 in 10 000 and it increases to 2 in 10 000 on HRT. So the risk is very small and remains very small on HRT. The risk is higher in those over 60 years of age, but HRT is rarely started in this age group. Smoking and being overweight increase the risk. Talk to your doctor about this, if you think that you may be at risk.

I'm fit and active with no risk factors for heart disease – will I benefit from HRT?

If you have no risks for heart disease, HRT will not improve this as your risk is very low anyway, but you may benefit from HRT by avoiding osteoporosis (thin bones). This is more common in slim women. HRT also helps to relieve hot flushes. Check with your doctor about the possibility of having a bone density scan if you think you may be at risk for osteoporosis.

From the point of view of heart health, who will benefit most from taking HRT?

No one.

I have been taking HRT for 7 years and I think that it is wonderful – I now feel a new woman! However, my doctor says that I should stop it soon. How long should I continue taking HRT?

HRT is usually taken for hot flushes for up to 5 years. Bone benefits continue on beyond 10 years, but the breast cancer risk increases. So, at present, we recommend HRT is stopped.

I'm on HRT at the moment. Do I need regular check-ups?

It is very important that you attend for regular check-ups at first every 3 months and then 6-monthly, and follow your doctor's instructions. For these check-ups, make a note of any queries or concerns that you might have and discuss them with your doctor.

I have been on oral HRT for some months and my doctor has arranged for me to have a lipid test. Why?

The doctor is checking to make sure that you are not at risk of heart disease, which is good medical practice. Up to the menopause, women usually have a raised high density lipoprotein level (HDL) (greater than 1.3) which helps protect them from coronary disease. This HDL gradually falls after the menopause unless HRT is taken. It is important that women should always have a 'full lipid profile' taken (HDL as well as LDL) because a high total cholesterol may reflect good

(HDL) rather than bad (LDL) cholesterol levels. Reducing your total cholesterol in this situation might reduce the protective HDL and be counter-productive.

A full lipid profile will also tell you about your triglycerides. Oral HRT can raise triglycerides, but HRT patches have no effect on triglyceride levels. A high triglyceride level is more of a risk in women than in men; the best means of lowering it is by weight loss and regular exercise, along with a low saturated fat diet. An underactive thyroid and too much alcohol can also be a cause.

I do find the advice on HRT confusing – can you clarify it for me?

I'll try, but doctors find it confusing too!

- HRT definitely helps menopausal symptoms, e.g. hot flushes.

- It definitely helps prevent thin bones (osteoporosis).

- It does not protect against heart disease developing.

- In those with coronary disease, it does not benefit them, so it is not a treatment for heart disease.

- In those with heart disease, it still helps menopausal symptoms and osteoporosis.

- HRT increases the risk of breast cancer.

- Overall, HRT is indicated only if menopausal symptoms are severe and intolerable. It is then given for as short a time as possible and at as low a dose as possible.

I'm concerned that my wife is at risk of heart disease and I want her to take it seriously; she smokes and is rather well padded! However, her doctor does not seem to be bothering either. What should I tell her?

You should point out that women are just as vulnerable to coronary disease as men. Some women don't recognise this and play down any symptoms of chest discomfort. They usually put their family first. Sometimes they might hide things from the doctor, which makes diagnosis difficult for both angina and a heart attack.

Your wife and every other woman should take heart disease seriously and her doctor, like all doctors, should recognise that women with a mixture of symptoms need taking seriously. Women may be reassured too easily because most women believe themselves to be less likely to have heart disease than men.

Post-menopausal women are at more risk and, even when the symptoms are not typical, these should be discussed and heart disease ruled in or out.

Women are just as likely as men to develop coronary disease if they smoke and just as likely to benefit if they stop. Keeping to a sensible weight and taking regular exercise are also important preventative measures. Tell her that heart disease is an equal opportunity killer and that she should do her best to avoid it for her sake and that of her family.

Send for the British Heart Foundation's booklet *Women and heart disease* and present it to her!

3 | Angina

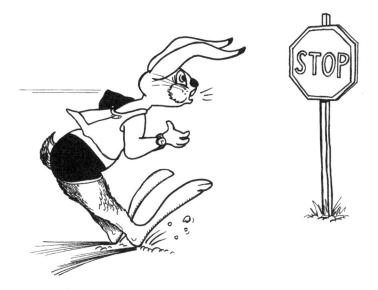

Each year in the UK around 320 000 people visit their doctor for angina. Over six million people in America and two million in the UK are affected. *Angina* (pronounced 'ann-jy-na') is a symptom of a problem, not a disease in itself. It is usually caused by narrowing of the coronary arteries by atheroma (see introduction to Chapter 2). It can also be caused by a high blood pressure (see the section **Risks of high blood pressure** in Chapter 2), disease of the aortic valve (see Chapter 7), severe anaemia, and rapid palpitations (see Chapter 6) or a mixture of conditions. Far and away the commonest cause is coronary artery disease (see Chapter 2).

The coronary arteries supply oxygen to the heart and the heart gets this supply between its beats, when it is refuelling itself. This means that the faster your heart beats, the less oxygen there is for the heart itself. If your arteries are narrowed, the flow is restricted. The balance will function well enough when you are not doing anything but, when your heart speeds up, there will come a point when the narrow arteries restrict the supply of oxygen to your heart muscle and pain develops. This is when angina is most often felt, as a chest pain, when you are active or when you are worked up about something, because the demands of your heart for oxygen are not being met by the supply of oxygenated blood to your heart muscle.

SYMPTOMS

My husband has got angina. He is obviously in pain but cannot describe it easily. What does it feel like?

The pain usually begins behind the breast bone. It is often felt as a tightness or a squeezing sensation; your husband probably describes it best by clenching his fist in front of his chest (see Figure 3.1).

The pain of angina can be regarded as a built-in warning device and tells him that the heart has reached its maximum workload. The onset of pain or discomfort indicates that he should slow down or stop any exertion. Alternatively, if emotion (such as anger) has lead to this, then he should relax and remove himself from the situation.

You *cannot* usually point to where angina pain is felt; it is more widespread and felt across the chest. It is brought on usually by effort, so it will build up if that effort is continued. When it begins, it is often quite mild – more of an ache – so it is easily confused with indigestion. Angina pain may spread (radiate) to the throat or neck, the jaw (like toothache), to the left or right arm or both, and sometimes to the back or stomach. It usually goes down the inside of the arm, in contrast to muscle pain which runs over the shoulder and down the outside of the arm. Rarely, angina occurs in one of these places without being in the chest; for example, a person gets pain in the left arm on effort which is relieved by resting.

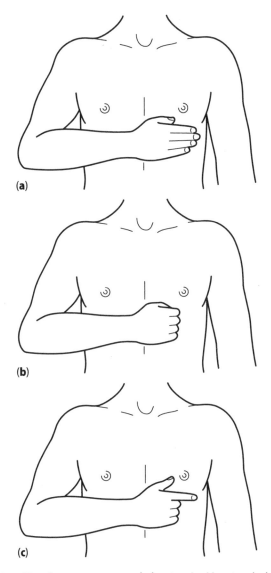

Figure 3.1 Hand movements and chest pain. Heart pain is usually described with the flat of the hand (**a**) or a clenched fist (**b**). Heart pain is almost never localised or pointed to (**c**).

Can my husband's chest pain be from causes other than heart disease?

There are many other causes of chest pain and here are some pointers to stop you worrying unnecessarily.

- *Joint or muscle pain* This is often worse when someone is changing position. This sort of pain can be reproduced by pressing on the ribs or breastbone.

- *Lung disorders* This pain is aggravated when you take a deep breath.

- *Stomach problems* Indigestion after a meal or on bending with an acid taste in your mouth (acid reflux).

- *Gallbladder problems* Colicky pain after a fatty meal may suggest gallstones.

- *Stress, anxiety* or *overbreathing.*

Nobody should have chest pain that is a mystery. Do not assume your husband has angina but also do not let him ignore the pain. Get him to ask his doctor's advice. Table 3.1 shows the main differences in signs between heart and not-heart pain.

What is the difference between angina and a heart attack?

Angina is the result of a temporary shortage of oxygen available to the heart muscle, usually caused by exercise or strong feelings. Angina pain usually passes off when you stop activity, or very shortly after taking a 'nitrate' tablet (see the section **Treatment** below). Angina results from narrowed coronary arteries.

A heart attack is different (see Chapter 4). The pain build-up is more severe, lasts longer and does not decrease when you stop any activity. It may be modified if you take nitrate tablets but is not relieved. You will often find that you sweat and you may feel sick. A heart attack is caused by an artery blocking off, usually when a clot forms on a narrowed area.

Table 3.1 Chest pain characteristics

Typical angina pain	*Not heart pain*
Tightness	Sharp (not severe)
Pressure	Knife-like
Weight on the chest	Stabbing
Heaviness	'Like a stitch'
Constriction – like a band	Shooting
Ache	Localised
Dull	Positional
Burning	Reproduced by pressure
Crushing	Located elsewhere than mid-chest
Retrosternal (behind breast bone)	Not exertional
Precipitated by exercise	Not relieved by GTN
and/or emotion	Relieved by antacids
Relieved promptly by GTN*	

*GTN, glyceryl trinitrate (see the section *Medication* later in this chapter)

I have been diagnosed as having unstable angina. What is this?

Angina that occurs more frequently with ever-decreasing activity is known as unstable angina. For example, if it is worse when you walk 22 metres (25 yards) rather than 0.8 km (half a mile). It may also occur at minimal activity or at rest, or wake you from sleep. You should see your doctor urgently if:

- you are getting angina for the first time;

- the pain is getting worse and occurring more frequently;

- the pain happens when you are not doing anything.

I am on medicine for angina and I still often get pains. If I get an attack of angina, it is difficult to know when I should bother the doctor. What should I do?

There are various instances when this would be advisable.

- If you have been newly diagnosed with angina and pain occurs when you are walking less than 22 metres (25 yards) on the flat.

- If it occurs at rest (usually in bed).

- If the pain lasts longer than 20 minutes in spite of nitrates (see below).

- If you are very breathless.

- If you feel faint or light-headed with the pain.

- If the pain comes on while you are convalescing from a recent heart attack.

When should I dial 999 rather than just call a doctor?

If the pain lasts longer than 20 minutes, in spite of nitrate tablets or spray, then dial 999. Tell them that you need an ambulance and have a 'possible heart attack'. Try another nitrate tablet or spray if the pain continues; crunch a 300 mg tablet of aspirin and then swallow it. Aspirin thins the blood and can help prevent unstable angina developing into a heart attack as well as limiting the damage a heart attack can do.

I have angina, but I want to live an active life. Is there any activity that is likely to bring my angina on?

Any form of exercise can bring angina on – climbing stairs, carrying shopping, walking up an incline and rushing. Angina may be more of a problem in cold or windy weather, or when you are carrying something heavy or going for a walk too soon after a large meal. It also occurs when you are under emotional stress, especially anger. It can vary a lot from day to day, but if it is becoming more frequent and the distances you can walk shorter, you should report back to your doctor.

I sometimes get a pain after eating. The doctor told me this was 'post-prandial angina'. What exactly is this?

As your doctor says, this is angina which occurs after a meal. Eating a large meal can increase the work that the heart has to do by 20% (to digest the food) so angina may occur if you have coronary narrowings. The usual sequence goes something like this: meal – walk the dog – angina. This happens because you have exercised too soon after a meal, adding stress to the heart. Post-prandial angina can be a warning of more severe coronary disease and I expect your doctor will be giving you some more tests.

Sometimes when I drive, for instance in the rush hour, I get angina symptoms – am I wise to carry on?

No. You must not drive until your symptoms are controlled, either by medication or surgery.

TESTS

What tests might I have to undergo for angina?

Your doctor will examine you, check your weight and blood pressure and listen to your heart for certain sounds and noises in your chest. Your blood should be checked when you have not eaten overnight to measure the fat content (cholesterol – see the section *Risks of high cholesterol levels* in Chapter 2).

Your doctor may want to do an *electrocardiogram* (ECG) (see below) which is a means of checking the way the heart works and whether there is any damage. An exercise electrocardiogram (see question below) on a treadmill machine or bicycle may be used to assess how well your heart behaves under stress and how much you can do.

Some people may be sent to a specialist heart doctor (a cardiologist) who may suggest that you have an *angiogram*, with a cardiac catheter inserted (see the section *Angiogram* below).

ECG

My doctor is sending me for an ECG next week. I am not sure what this involves – will it mean time in hospital for an operation?

No, and it is painless and takes only 10 minutes to do. An electro-cardiogram (ECG in the UK, EKG in Europe or the USA) is a simple painless test which looks at the electrical activity of the heart. It tells the doctor about your heart rate, whether you are likely to have a heart attack and if you have any hardening of your arteries, and whether your heart's rhythm is regular or not.

You will have electrodes (usually sticky pads) applied to your arms and legs, and six are placed across your chest (see Figure 3.2) to record the electrical activity in your heart, while you are not doing anything. Men with hairy chests may need a small area shaved. The resulting ECG trace gives an electrical picture of your heart. It is not dangerous and you cannot be electrocuted!

What does an exercise ECG involve?

An exercise ECG records the electrical activity of your heart when you are walking on a treadmill (or bicycle) exercise machine (see Figure 3.3); in other words, it imitates you walking in the street or uphill, when the effect of any coronary narrowing is most likely to show up. It is used to help your doctor when unsure whether you have angina or, if you have angina, to decide whether it is severe or not.

The test speeds up every 3 minutes and the uphill slope is increased to give your heart a gradual stress. The doctor looks for any changes on the ECG, whether you are getting chest pains or are unduly short of breath, and an eye is kept on your blood pressure. Whilst on the treadmill, tell the doctor or technician if you have any pain or discomfort, or if you feel light-headed or sweaty. When the machine is stopped, the heart rate is monitored for another 5 minutes or so to see what happens.

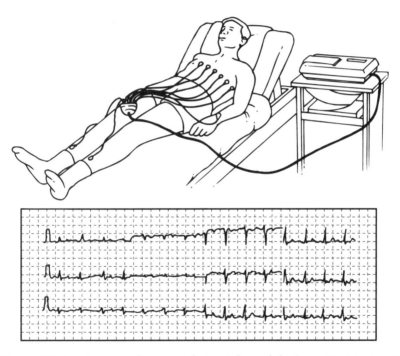

Figure 3.2 An electrocardiogram is being taken while the patient is at rest. The trace from the machine is also shown.

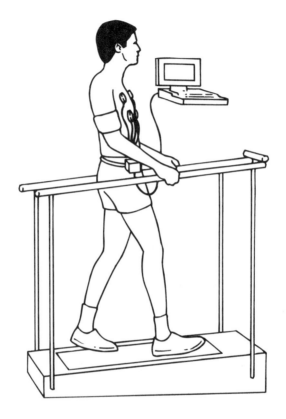

Figure 3.3 An electrocardiogram is being taken while the patient is on a treadmill.

I have an appointment for an exercise ECG. How should I prepare for it?

Wear comfortable shoes and loose clothing. Do not eat a meal or have caffeine drinks for 2 hours beforehand. Bring along any medication you are taking, including your nitrate tablets (see the section *Treatment* on p. 99). If you have a cold or flu, tell your doctor so that the test can be postponed.

My ECG last week was absolutely normal. However, because the doctor still thinks that I have angina, I have got to go for more tests. Why?

You probably had an ECG at rest (lying down) and, if this was normal, it does not rule out coronary artery disease. It can be falsely reassuring, so an exercise ECG is usually advised. If the ECG is abnormal at rest or on exercise, you may then need further tests to try and find out if coronary narrowing exists and how severe it is.

What makes the exercise test abnormal?

An exercise test may suggest that you have coronary artery disease if the ECG changes, if you get pain of a certain kind or get out of breath, or if your blood pressure falls. As a rule, the longer you can keep going, the better: 9 minutes is average and 12 minutes or more is good. The doctor will tell you the result of the test in the clinic and may make recommendations for treatment or further tests. If you get pain or your ECG shows changes in less than 6 minutes, then this is a strong sign that you have narrowed arteries and need specialised treatment.

My doctor says the exercise test is equivocal, so he can't be sure if there is or isn't a problem, and is sending me for a nuclear scan. Will I be radioactive?

No, but I understand your concern. A 'nuclear' or perfusion scan is an outpatient test which looks at blood flow to the heart. If there is an area of the heart muscle that does not show up on the scan, it could be a permanent scar such as occurs after a heart attack. If an area does not show up after exercise but returns a few hours later, it means the blood supply to that area is reduced by a narrowing in the coronary artery and there is only temporary lack of blood nutrients, so the heart muscle is viable and it is not a scar.

A nuclear scan is used to clarify any doubts when the ECG alone gives an uncertain result. It can also be used when people can't exercise (for example, because they have arthritis), when the heart can be speeded up using drugs through a vein in the arm. A scan like this helps the doctor decide what's best for you and there is no need to be worried about it.

Angiogram

I have been told to go to the hospital for an angiogram. What is this and what does it involve?

A coronary angiogram (pronounced 'ann-gee-o-gram') is also known as cardiac catheterisation. This is a technique for establishing if there are any narrowings in your coronary arteries, how severe they are and whether they represent an increased risk of heart attack (see Figure 3.4). If narrowings are severe and in dangerous places, the doctor will then know that surgery is the best treatment for you. An angiogram can also give information about the heart valves and the quality of the muscle pump (left ventricle) and whether there is any damage.

The test involves small tubes (catheters) being passed through your arteries. Special X-rays are then taken of the coronary arteries and the heart muscle. When a dye is injected into the tube, any narrowings will be shown and any danger discovered. This test is straightforward but only done when there is a probability of narrowing that could be corrected by an operation or by the technique of *angioplasty* (see question later on *Percutaneous transluminal coronary angioplasty*).

You will usually be in and out the same day. You will be given a ward bed and have nothing to eat or drink for 4 hours before the test as, just occasionally, the dye used to show up the arteries can make people feel sick.

You may be given medicine to help you relax. You will be taken to the catheter laboratory usually by a porter or a nurse. Some hospitals use trolleys, others wheelchairs and, in many, you simply walk down with the nurse. The laboratory nurses will introduce themselves and you will meet the cardiologist who is doing the angiogram. The 'cath

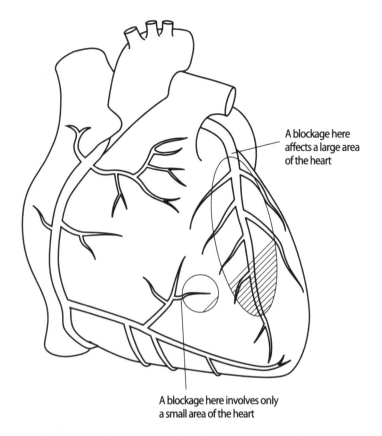

A blockage here affects a large area of the heart

A blockage here involves only a small area of the heart

Figure 3.4 The relative risks of coronary artery blockage.

lab' is full of sophisticated equipment all designed to help diagnose your problem.

You will be asked to lie on a table (usually it is rather hard!) beneath an X-ray camera, which will make a noise when in use. TV screens will show the procedure as it's happening, so that you can watch what's going on (if you want to).

There are two ways of doing the angiogram – one from the arm and one from the leg. Most procedures are done from the leg, but different hospitals have different procedures, and the leg procedure may not be suitable for some people because of hardened leg arteries.

A local anaesthetic is applied to the top of your leg and you will feel a needle prick followed by a stinging numbing sensation. This is the only discomfort that you should feel. A fine tube is passed through the artery all the way to your heart. You will not feel this tube. Once the tube (the catheter) is safely in place, dye is injected into the arteries and the ventricle (pumping chamber) and pictures will be taken. You will hear the camera run several times as pictures are taken from different angles, and the camera will move over your chest to the left and right. Imagine your arteries to the heart are like a big tree and that you are walking around the bottom looking up at all the big and little branches; as you move around, any area of overlap becomes clear. So it is with the camera: it moves to unravel the branches so that nothing is missed. You may be asked to hold your breath from time to time and your arms may be put over your head if they are in the camera's way.

The whole procedure usually takes less than 30 minutes and often only 10–15 minutes.

I am told I need an angiogram but I saw on TV a new kind of angiogram using CT scanning. What's this?

It's known as 64-channel multi-detector computed tomography (MDCT). It is an outpatient specialised X-ray procedure which can take pictures of your arteries in less than half an hour. You have an injection in a vein (not an artery) and your heart is slowed, usually by taking a beta-blocker drug beforehand, as this leads to better pictures. It's an exciting new technique which does not replace an angiogram but can be used instead when the diagnosis of heart disease is unlikely but the doctor is not certain. It also is used when the person is at risk but has no symptoms – for example, someone with diabetes who has no chest pain but an abnormal ECG. It does involve X-rays so cannot be used casually in a check-up. New scanners are being introduced which are claimed to reduce X-ray exposure by 80% so this is going to be an exciting area of development with the possibility of repeated scans to monitor progress.

MRI does not involve X-rays so can I have an MRI instead of an angiogram?

Not yet. Magnetic resonance arteriography (MRA) can show up any problems in the aorta and renal (kidney) arteries but not yet in the coronary arteries. Magnetic resonance imaging (MRI) can tell us about the structure and pumping of the heart.

Is there any difference between an angiogram from the arm or the leg?

The leg approach does not involve stitches but pressure is needed for 10 minutes or so to stop the bleeding (a tiny hole is made in the artery by a fine needle). To prevent re-bleeding, you will be advised to rest in bed for 4–6 hours. This technique is 'percutaneous' which means 'through the skin' but no surgical cut is involved. Devices have been developed to 'plug' the hole in the artery and, if you are a suitable candidate, the artery will be closed and you will not need pressure on the groin. You will rest in bed for about an hour and then get up and about, going home sooner.

The arm approach is usually percutaneous at the wrist (radial artery) and does not need bed or chair rest for more than an hour.

The arm approach at the elbow can be percutaneous but often needs a cut and then stitches (the jargon we use is cut-down). Again, you are up and moving very soon. The wrist and leg techniques are the most common. The wrist approach is being used more frequently but is not suitable for everyone.

*I have been on warfarin tablets for some time now, to prevent
blood clots. Do I need to stop or reduce my warfarin before the
angiogram?*

Warfarin is a medication used to prevent blood clots from forming.
It is not always necessary to stop or reduce warfarin with an
angiogram taken from the arm, but it is essential with the leg approach
to prevent severe bruising. We usually advise four days of no therapy
before an angiogram. Always remind the doctor that you are taking
warfarin so your clotting can be checked before the procedure.

*I'm taking aspirin every day – do I need to stop this for the
angiogram?*

No, this is not necessary. The mild blood-thinning action of aspirin
helps prevent clotting in the artery narrowings but it does not
usually significantly increase the tendency to bruising or bleeding. The
same applies if you are taking clopidogrel as an alternative to aspirin,
or both together.

Is the angiogram at all painful?

The only discomfort should be the injection of local anaesthetic.
When the dye is injected into your muscle pump, you may feel hot
and flushed with a strange warm feeling in your bottom. This passes
quickly. Sometimes, when the catheter is in the pumping chamber,
your heart may appear to miss a beat or flutter for a few seconds. Don't
be afraid; this is all routine.

After the procedure, pressure will be applied to your groin to stop
the bleeding (about 15 minutes) and you will be asked to rest in bed
for 4–6 hours while the small hole in your artery closes. If your arm
has been used, a pressure bandage will be applied to your wrist.

Is the angiogram procedure dangerous?

All tests have a slight risk but in an experienced centre the complication rate is about 1 in 1000. Remember that this figure includes emergency cases and people who are ill as well as people undergoing routine tests. The test is never done without a good reason and the risks are very low.

What happens after I have had my angiogram?

Most departments have a recovery area, but if this is not available your ward nurse will collect you from the 'cath' department and take you back to your bed on the ward. If you have had an angiogram by the leg approach, until you are safely back in bed, you may be asked to press on the leg used and to keep it as straight as possible. This is to prevent further bleeding from the site. This rarely happens but, if it does, don't panic; press as the nurse or doctor did and call for help.

Your nurse will record your pulse and blood pressure at frequent intervals to check that all is well. The site of the catheter insertion will be checked and the pulses felt in your feet or arm. If you notice any blood, apply pressure as before and tell your nurse. If your arm or leg feels cold, also tell the nurse.

If the arm has been used, you will get up almost straight away but, if the leg is used or a 'plug' has not been inserted, you will be asked to remain in bed for 4–6 hours, still keeping that leg straight. When you wish to go to the toilet, the nurse will bring the urinal or bedpan. If you have had a leg angiogram, you can usually get out of bed after 4–6 hours (1–2 hours if a plug has been inserted). Check when it is safe to get up. Don't get up without checking first.

How long after my angiogram will I get my results?

When your films have been developed and studied, the doctors will come to discuss the results of your angiogram with you, usually the same day. Some hospitals have a weekly conference so there may be a delay. Any further treatment that you may need, either medical or surgical, will then be discussed with you, either before you go home or in the outpatient clinic after the conference.

If the coronary arteries are hardened, the doctor will be able to show you your results by means of a diagram.

What happens after I have been discharged from hospital, following the angiogram?

Problems are rare. Sometimes the leg is bruised but this slowly fades over 2–3 weeks. Occasionally a hard lump, like a gland, is felt in the groin: this is just a bruise again. Don't worry – if it is tender, take painkillers. Have a quiet evening when you get home, but you can be up and about the next day. Any sticking plaster is best removed in the bath the following morning. If you have had a leg angiogram, you should avoid strenuous exercise for 48 hours. If you have had an arm cut-down angiogram, you need to make arrangements for stitch removal if the non-dissolvable sort have been used – your family doctor will do this at about seven days. If pain continues, or the scar looks red and swollen, go to your doctor. It is unusual, but infection can occur and antibiotics will then be needed.

If you are taking warfarin, you should start your tablets again the same day, although it is a good plan to confirm this with the hospital doctor before leaving. Those who work can get back to work usually in a couple of days; driving is possible also the next day.

I always thought that angina was a man's problem. Do women get angina?

Coronary disease is the most important cause of death and disability in women. It is seven times more likely to cause premature death in women than breast cancer. Angina is just as much a woman's problem as a man's (see the section **Women and coronary artery disease** in Chapter 2).

I have had my angiogram and my arteries are clear, but I still have angina. My doctor says that I have Syndrome X – what does this mean?

This is a condition which is more common in women. There is no extra risk of a heart attack or dropping dead, but nearly two-thirds of people with chest pain and normal arteries who suffer from angina are significantly limited by it. It is very difficult to treat. Drugs that relax the arteries to try and improve the blood flow (nitrates, calcium antagonists, nicorandil) may help. It is important to rule out other problems that may mimic angina, in particular a hiatus hernia or excess stomach acid.

People who suffer from Syndrome X can help themselves by:

- not smoking;

- exercising as much as possible; and

- losing weight if they need to.

It is a very frustrating condition to treat and we do not have all the answers – some people are helped, some are not. It is important, however, not to give up trying to help. It is a real condition and not 'in the mind'.

TREATMENT

What is there, apart from medication, to treat angina?

Relief measures other than medication include angioplasty and surgery. First, there are some general self-help measures. These have been discussed before but to summarise:

- stop smoking;

- lose weight;

- cut down on alcohol;

- take exercise;
- Take life easier by reducing stress.

Table 3.2 Drugs for angina

Generic name	Trade name
Nitrates	
Isosorbide mononitrate	Elantan, Imdur, Ismo, Isotard
Glyceryl trinitrate (tablets or spray)	
Beta blockers	
Atenolol	Tenormin, Totamol
Acebutolol	Sectral
Bisoprolol	Monocor, Emcor
Metoprolol	Betaloc, Lopresor
Nadolol	Corgard
Oxprenolol	Trasicor
Pindolol	Visken
Propranolol	Inderal, Beta-Prograne
Timolol	Betim, Blocadren
Calcium antagonists	
Amlodipine	Istin
Diltiazem	Adizem, Dilzem, Tildiem
Felodipine	Plendil
Nicardipine	Cardene
Nifedipine	Adalat, Adalat LA, Cardilate MR, Coracten XL
Nisoldipine	Syscor MR
Verapamil	Cordilox, Securon, Univer
Potassium channel activators	
Nicorandil	Ikorel
Sinus node slowers	
Ivabradine	Procoralan

The use of aspirin as a preventative drug has been discussed a lot in the media recently. What does aspirin do?

Aspirin helps stop blood clotting. It reduces by 25% the risk of a heart attack and helps prevent strokes in people with angina or who have had a heart attack. You only need 75 mg a day and should not take more, unless specified by your doctor; 75 mg is a quarter of an adult 300 mg tablet. It occasionally upsets the stomach and a small number of people with asthma or bronchitis may be sensitive to it (it worsens the wheezing). Overall it is cheap, safe and very effective. Special types of coated aspirin are available for those who get indigestion but they are not always helpful. Taking a compound like Alka-Seltzer is another way of taking aspirin and reducing the chances of a stomach upset; it contains 324 mg aspirin, so you will need to take only a quarter.

I get indigestion on aspirin – is there an alternative?

Clopidogrel (Plavix) 75 mg daily thins the blood to the same degree as aspirin and is used as an alternative. It is only available on prescription. It still may cause indigestion and it may be best to stay on aspirin and use a drug that blocks stomach acid such as omeprazole.

Medication

What relieves the pain of angina? Do I have to take medication?

Angina is relieved after 1–2 minutes by slowing down or stopping activity, or using a nitrate tablet or spray, usually GTN, short for glyceryl trinitrate. If you get pain on walking after a meal and stop to take an indigestion tablet, it will seem as if the tablet has helped. In fact it was the stopping that relieved the pain: this is often how angina and indigestion get confused.

Several drugs are available to stop angina occurring or to deal with an attack. We have already discussed cholesterol-lowering diets and tablets in Chapter 2 and it is essential that people with angina have a cholesterol test and know the result.

Anyone with angina should be prescribed and told how to use sublingual (under the tongue) nitrates and aspirin or clopidogrel. The other medications – oral nitrates, beta-blockers, calcium antagonists and potassium channel activators (discussed below) – are prescribed as necessary. See Table 3.2 for a list of currently available medications. Check the trade name against the generic name.

Nitrates

How do the nitrates work?

Nitrates open up the arteries by relaxing the muscle in the artery wall. They relax the coronary arteries to improve the blood flow; by relaxing the peripheral arteries (such as in the legs) and veins, they reduce the work the heart has to do. As the problem is one of too much demand and too little supply, nitrates attempt to rectify the situation by improving supply (by dilating the artery) and reducing demand (the heart pumps against less resistance as the arteries are relaxed).

My mother has been given sublingual nitrates but seems unclear what to do. As I am her carer, what do I need to know?

Sublingual nitrates are taken in tablet or spray form and are absorbed via the veins under the tongue. They are effective in 1–2 minutes and last 20–30 minutes. They relieve attacks and can be used when your mother fears an attack; for example, she can use them at the bottom of a hill before she starts to climb. Headache is the main side effect.

After you collect them from the chemist, the tablets last only about 8 weeks and have to be stored correctly.

- Keep the tablets in the airtight bottle in which they have been dispensed.

- After use, close the bottle tightly.

- Do not put cotton wool, other tablets, or anything else in the bottle with these tablets.

- Store the tablets in a cool place. When your mother carries them with her, tell her not to put them too close to the heat of her body – she could keep them in a purse or handbag (other people can carry them in a briefcase).

- If she does not use the tablets within 8 weeks of opening the bottle, get a fresh supply and discard the old tablets. An active tablet produces a slight burning sensation when placed under the tongue. If this does not happen, you should get a fresh supply for her.

The spray lasts 2–3 years but is more expensive. It is useful when attacks are infrequent as it lasts longer in storage. Tablets can be bought over the counter without prescription whereas the spray needs a doctor's prescription.

I have been given nitrate tablets to swallow. Are these different from the sublingual ones?

Yes, nitrates also come as tablets that are swallowed once or twice daily and can be taken on a regular basis to reduce your angina attacks and improve your ability to take exercise. The commonest are isosorbide mononitrate which are taken twice daily, or in slow release formulations (Imdur, Elantan, Ismo) once daily. They must not be taken more often or the body gets used to them – known as tolerance – and they are then ineffective in relieving angina. Sublingual tablets are only taken when you have, or fear, an angina attack coming on.

There are also nitrate patches which are effective when placed on the skin like a plaster; they have to be taken off after 12 hours or your body again develops tolerance. Used 12 hours on and 12 hours off, they act as a back-up and can be helpful overnight if put on in the evening and taken off in the morning. They should not be used on their own because, with 12 hours off, no angina protection is provided for that period.

> *Since I have been taking nitrates for my angina, I seem to get headaches. Is this due to my medication and are there any other side effects?*

Headache is certainly the most frequent side effect. Occasionally you may get palpitations (see Chapter 6) or flushing and sometimes the tablets under your tongue make your breath smell. Rarely, and particularly if the tablets are taken within a short while of drinking alcohol or when starving, you might get a dizzy attack, caused by a temporary lowering of blood pressure. If headaches are a problem, the nitrates will be stopped and other drugs substituted.

Beta-blockers

> *I have been prescribed beta-blockers for my angina. What are these?*

These are very important medications. They are the only ones (besides aspirin, cholesterol-lowering tablets and ACE inhibitors) that have been medically proved to lengthen the life of many people with heart problems. Beta-blockers reduce the work that the heart has to do by slowing the heart rate and lowering the blood pressure. They also reduce the force with which the heart muscle contracts, so that it needs less energy. By slowing the heart rate, they allow more time for blood to flow to the heart past the narrowings, and they blunt the heart rate's response to exercise. If you were to run for a bus, your heart rate might rise to 130 beats per minute (bpm); with a beta-blocker it might not get above 110 bpm, so you would be less likely to develop angina. A slower heart rate is therefore a feature of beta-blocker treatment and one of the main reasons that they are so effective in reducing the number of attacks that people experience, as well as allowing them to walk further. They also help people to live longer after a heart attack and may therefore help protect people with angina from serious complications.

Beta-blockers are swallowed, once or twice daily. The commonest in use are atenolol and bisoprolol but a large number exist. They should never be stopped suddenly because the heart can rebound the other way, and this can lead to severe bouts of chest pain or even a heart attack.

I have been taking beta-blockers regularly. Are there any side effects with this treatment?

Yes, beta-blockers can cause:

- wheezing (they should not be given to asthmatics);

- breathlessness and fatigue (general tiredness with feelings of being 'worn out' or 'washed out');

- cold hands and feet and heavy leg muscles (by slowing the circulation);

- muzzy head with poor concentration and vivid dreams;

- rarely, depression;

- occasional erection problems in men and reduced sex drive in women.

Do not stop taking your medication if you experience any of these effects. Tell your doctor and your tablets can be changed.

I have been very forgetful lately. Do you think this could be due to the beta-blockers I am taking? Are there any others I could take?

Yes. Some beta-blockers (such as atenolol) are soluble in water and do not cross into the brain, so dreams and confusion or forgetfulness are less common. These are known as hydrophilic (dissolve in water) types. Others (such as propranolol) are soluble in fat (lipophilic) and can cross into the brain. Although you may have more side effects with propranolol, you may also find that you are less anxious.

I have noticed that I have a slight tremor. Can beta-blockers relieve tremor and shakiness?

Yes, beta-blockers can be very effective, particularly propranolol, if you have tremor. As a result they can also help people with Parkinson's disease. It is also claimed that they improve the performance of snooker players and golfers! This is likely where anxiety and tremor are a major problem, of course, but the routine use of beta-blockers to improve performance is not approved of!

If my pulse drops below 50, should I stop taking my beta-blockers?

No. Beta-blockers act to slow the heart. The coronary arteries receive their oxygen and food between the beats, so the slower the rate, the more time the heart has to receive its food supply.
Your treatment will only be stopped if, owing to your slow heart rate, your symptoms of lethargy and fatigue become a problem. It is best to reduce the dose first. Do not stop any treatment without your doctor's advice. Beta-blockers should certainly not be stopped suddenly as this can cause a rebound chest pain and could be very dangerous.

When is the best time to take beta-blockers?

The once-a-day variety such as atenolol or bisoprolol are useful for people who have problems in remembering to take tablets (see question later in this section), and these are often best taken at night. This is a useful time to take them if they make you feel drowsy.

Is it a disaster if I forget to collect my prescription and run out of tablets?

You must try not to run out of your tablets as you may get rebound chest pain. Your chemist will give you some until you get your prescription renewed: it is dangerous to stop beta-blockers suddenly (see question above about stopping tablets suddenly).

My doctor prescribed beta-blockers some time ago and now has put me on nitrates as well. Is this safe?

Yes, the combination is very effective. For example, you may be given atenolol plus isosorbide mononitrate.

Calcium antagonists

What are calcium antagonists (calcium blockers)?

Calcium is an ion (an electrically charged particle) which increases the tone of muscles and strengthens the contraction of the muscle. The muscle in the wall of the artery depends on calcium for its tone, so if the movement of calcium into the muscle cell is 'antagonised' or 'blocked', the muscle will relax. As the muscle relaxes the artery becomes bigger, blood flow increases and the demands on the heart decrease.

Do calcium antagonists act in the same way as nitrates?

In a way, yes. They both increase the size of arteries but by different mechanisms. In combination they may have an additive effect, so you may be prescribed both.

Can I take calcium antagonists with beta-blockers?

Only some calcium antagonists. Verapamil must never be taken with a beta-blocker because of the danger of slowing the heart too dramatically. Diltiazem is used cautiously by some hospitals. Amlodipine, felodipine and nifedipine are quite safe and effective in combination with beta-blockers. Never mix your medications without first checking with your doctor or pharmacist.

I have not got on well with verapamil so my doctor plans to change my medication to nifedipine. Are there differences between the various types of calcium antagonists?

There are several calcium antagonists on the market and they have some differences which are important. Verapamil and diltiazem slow the heart rate as well as widening blood vessels, so they are a good alternative to beta-blockers, if beta-blockers are not suitable for you (for instance if you have asthma) or they are giving you unacceptable side effects. The calcium antagonists amlodipine, felodipine and nifedipine do not slow your heart rate and are often used in combination with beta-blockers.

Will I experience any side effects with calcium antagonists?

There are plenty of calcium antagonists on the market, so if you are prescribed one that does not suit you, tell your doctor so that your medication can be changed. Two common effects you are likely to experience are headaches and flushing, because these medications open up the arteries.

Another common side effect is swollen ankles and this does not respond to water tablets (diuretics; see the section *Treatment* in Chapter 5). Ankle swelling may improve as the dose is decreased but often the tablets have to be discontinued. Verapamil and diltiazem are less likely to lead to swollen ankles.

Constipation can be a problem if you are taking verapamil (and more so the older you get). High-fibre diets and lactulose can help but, if constipation becomes a serious problem, your doctor will change you onto another type of calcium antagonist.

Rarely, eye pain and gum problems occur. Calcium antagonists do not usually cause the tiredness that can be a problem with beta-blockers. They may be less effective if you continue to smoke, whereas beta-blocker treatment is not affected by smoking. (Remember smoking causes heart attacks and can kill you.)

Why did my doctor prescribe beta-blockers for me rather than calcium antagonists?

Usually calcium antagonists are prescribed only if beta-blockers are not suitable or are giving side effects. Some calcium antagonists can be combined with beta-blockers to give an additional benefit and all of them can be combined with nitrates (see question above about combining these medications).

I have found that beta-blockers have given me an unfortunate problem, in affecting my love life. My doctor says he will try me on calcium antagonists, but not straight away. Why not?

Your doctor will do this gradually. The beta-blocker must be wound down and the calcium antagonist wound up over a period of time. Calcium antagonists do not give you protection when beta-blockers are suddenly stopped.

Potassium channel activators

> *I seem to have been given all sorts of medication for my angina over time. My doctor has now said he wants me to try a new type called a potassium channel activator. I have never heard of this one! Will it do any good?*

These are medications which work half like a nitrate and half like a calcium antagonist. There is only one available at the moment – nicorandil. It can be used on its own or in combination with the other three types of medication for angina (see Table 3.2). It does not cause swollen ankles, but headaches can be a problem. It is as good as the other medications but not any better, and it is very expensive in comparison. It tends to be used after the other options have been tried and in this way can be very helpful. So if you have tried all the other options, you might – with luck – find that this suits you. Do not drive or operate machinery until settled on nicorandil and your performance is not impaired.

> *My doctor says she would like to try me on ivabradine as I have side effects on atenolol. How is it different?*

Ivabradine (Procoralan) is a new drug which slows the heart rate by an electrical action, so it is different from a beta-blocker. It may be used when beta-blockers are not tolerated and when the heart rhythm is regular (in sinus rhythm). Side effects are not common but include temporary visual disturbances (blurring), headache and dizziness. The pulse must be monitored to make sure it's regular and not below 50 beats per minute. Unlike beta-blockers there is no evidence to date that it prolongs life, but it does relieve angina pain.

Taking your medication

I am rather confused over the various medications available for angina. How many can I take at any one time?

Quite often, too many are taken at any one time! You will need aspirin and, usually, a cholesterol-lowering tablet (usually a statin) to reduce your chances of the coronary narrowings becoming worse. If one angina drug doesn't work, there is a tendency among doctors to add other medications rather than change the combination. If one drug partly works, it makes sense to increase its strength or add another in but, if it's not working, it makes no sense to continue it. There is no medical evidence that taking more than two medications for angina is better than one or two used properly. Many people could have their medication simplified, and it is possible that your doctor does not know exactly what you are taking, so always take all your tablets with you when you visit the surgery. If you are on many different tablets, discuss their strengths with your doctor and whether all of them are necessary. Do not make changes on your own. Many medications, taken twice or three times a day, are now in once-a-day formulations which makes life easier.

I am bad at remembering to take tablets. What should I do?

If you are on frequent doses (say three times a day), ask for a once-a-day alternative. For example, if you are on diltiazem 60 mg three times a day and isosorbide mononitrate 20 mg twice a day (five tablets), this could be changed to long-acting diltiazem 200 mg once a day and long-acting mononitrate once a day (that is, two tablets altogether) with the same effect. Beta-blockers are often best taken at night. Any sedative side effects can then be slept off.

Try to establish a routine. Take your medication at the same time of day – with your morning cup of tea or after brushing your teeth. If you are on a lot of tablets, special pill boxes are available, such as the Dosette, that are split into time of day and days of the week: ask your pharmacist about these. Ask your partner or friends to remind you or stick reminders by the phone or on the fridge (use one of those reminder magnets).

Remember not to run out (see a previous question on this). If you have a question about your medication, write it down – most people forget when they go to the doctor. It's a good idea to ask what each tablet is for and when you should take it. And remember to take all your tablets with you to the surgery – the doctor may not know what you are taking.

If you miss a dose of beta-blockers, take an extra tablet to catch up – others do not need boosting so just get back on schedule.

I have been told that cold remedies react with angina tablets. What can I do if I need them?

Some of these medications react, some don't. Show your heart tablets to the pharmacist and ask for advice about what you can or cannot take.

Am I allowed to drink alcohol with the medication?

Yes. However, alcohol does widen blood vessels, so the effects may add up with those of nitrates and calcium antagonists to give you more chance of a headache.

Are there any special dietary precautions that I should take while I am on angina medications?

The only precaution is to avoid grapefruit juice as it reacts with some medications in the liver – especially calcium antagonists and some statins. Advice on orange juice is to avoid it within 4 hours of taking your medication.

Are there any new medications for angina in the pipeline?

There are always new ones coming along. Most are variations on what we have already. We always need to see whether they are better than what we have or whether they can be added in to improve what we have. Always beware of exaggerated claims and look carefully at any statistics that are given.

I have heard that a drug called trimetazidine is available – what is this?

Trimetazidine is an interesting drug; it acts to improve oxygen supply by affecting how the cells of the heart work. It does not affect heart rate or blood pressure. It is not available (unless specially requested) in the UK but it is widely available elsewhere. It is an effective drug with minimal indigestion side effects and can be combined with all the other drugs available. It is the first of a class of drugs known as 'metabolic agents' because of its action improving how the cells function.

I read in the paper that there is a new drug called ranolozine about to become available – in what way is it different?

Ranolozine (Ranexa) acts a bit like trimetazidine (see above) but also inhibits the build-up of sodium and calcium in the cells, causing relaxation and improving oxygen supply, so angina is reduced. It can be added to other drugs but caution is needed in case there is a clash in the way they are metabolised (broken down). It can cause constipation, nausea and dizziness but these side effects are not common. Some evidence exists that it improves diabetic control. It appears to be a useful new therapy with a good safety profile.

Surgery

Angioplasty

> **I have been told that I need an angioplasty. What is this?**

Percutaneous transluminal coronary angioplasty (PTCA) is a method of using a balloon to squash or push the arterial narrowings out of the way. (The medical word for these narrowings is stenosis, pronounced 'sten-oh-siss'.) PTCA is often shortened to 'angioplasty'. Because stents are used in nearly all cases (see later) we often call this percutaneous coronary intervention (PCI).

It is performed in the catheter laboratory usually by the same team who does the angiograms (see the section *Angiograms* above) so you may meet some familiar faces. The doctor doing the operation will be the cardiologist, with whom you may already have had a consultation.

After a local anaesthetic, a thin tube (the catheter) is inserted into your artery at the top of your leg, or occasionally in an artery in your arm either at the elbow (brachial artery) or, more frequently, the wrist (radial artery). The catheter is guided under X-ray control to the heart, up the main artery known as the aorta (see Chapter 1). You cannot feel the tube moving. It is then directed into the coronary artery that contains the narrowing. This catheter is called the guide catheter (see Figure 3.5). A very fine wire (the guidewire) is now passed up through this catheter and into the coronary artery where it is steered past the narrowing. This may be a bit fiddly. Once it is across the narrowing, the balloon catheter is passed along the wire (like a monorail) and, following the wire, it slides across the narrowing. The balloon is blown up (inflated) once it is in position. This may cause some chest pain – let the doctor know if you have any pain at all.

The pressure in the balloon is increased and the narrowed part is pushed back into the wall of the artery where it has come from. The result is checked after the balloon has been deflated and removed back into the guide catheter. At this point the wire is still in place so that the

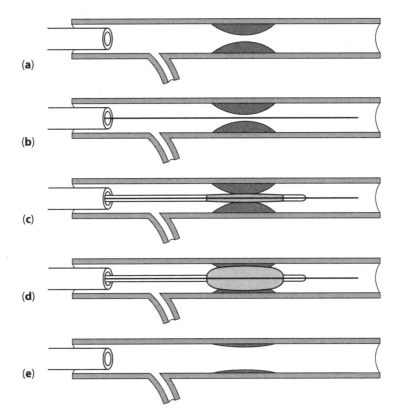

Figure 3.5 The technique of angioplasty. (**a**) Guide catheter in left coronary artery. (**b**) Guidewire advanced through narrowing. (**c**) Balloon positioned with markers. (**d**) Balloon inflated. (**e**) Catheter, with guidewire and balloon, removed leaving expanded artery.

balloon can be used again, or exchanged for a bigger balloon, if the result needs to be improved.

Once the doctor is satisfied with the result, the balloon and wire are removed; and you will be given a dye injection which checks how well the operation has gone; the guide catheter is then removed.

A small insertion sheath is left in the groin for about four hours, because the effects of blood thinning medication (heparin), used to prevent clotting on the wire or balloon, need to wear off. The sheath is removed on the ward and the groin pressed firmly for 20 minutes or so. If the radial artery (at the wrist) is used, it is firmly bandaged. A pressure device may be used which is slowly deflated. Often, the leg artery is plugged so that you can get up and about more quickly.

I am rather worried about the PTCA procedure. Will I be given any relaxing medicine beforehand?

This depends on you and how you are feeling. If you are anxious, then an injection of diazepam (Diazemuls or Valium) or midazolam helps you to relax.

Will I feel any pain when I undergo PTCA?

The local anaesthetic stings rather like when you have an angiogram. When the balloon is inflated, it blocks the artery temporarily (usually for 30 seconds or so), so you may get some chest pain. Let the doctor know if you are feeling any pain.

How long does the PTCA procedure last? Will I need to be in hospital for long?

Some procedures are quick (5–10 minutes), others take up to 1 hour. It depends on the number of narrowings in your particular case, whether they can be reached easily and whether you need a stent (see questions below on stents) or not.

Usually you will be in hospital for one night. This is the big advantage over bypass surgery (see the question later on bypass surgery) – you don't have to spend long in hospital and you recuperate rapidly.

How long will the effects of PTCA last?

In 7 cases out of 10, PTCA gives a complete cure. However, for reasons we don't understand fully, 30% of the narrowings come back in about 4–6 months. You will only know that the operation has not been entirely successful because your angina will return.

If my angina returns, can the PTCA be repeated?

Yes – up to five or six times, and each time it is performed, you have a 7 out of 10 chance of it remaining successful.

If you have no angina after 6 months, the effects will last for years, so the first 6 months constitute an important hurdle to overcome.

Can the cardiologist perform PTCA on more than one narrowing at a time?

Yes, as many as are necessary (but see the question below on unsuitable narrowings). Sometimes the procedure may be staged so that you come back for other narrowings to be done on a separate occasion. This decision depends on the importance of each narrowing and whether the procedure was an emergency or not – in an emergency only the most dangerous narrowing is done (the culprit), and the rest are completed when matters have settled down.

I am worried that things may go wrong when I have my PTCA. Is this likely?

Things are very unlikely to go wrong but, if they do not work out, there are other ways to sort out the problem. Complications are not common but they do occur. Sometimes the artery tears and closes completely. We can correct this by inserting a stent or moving on to bypass surgery (see below). However, angioplasty is successful over 95% of the time. You will be asked to sign a form giving your consent to having a stent inserted or bypass surgery, just in case the PTCA is not successful.

I have been told that I am not suitable for PTCA. Why is this?

Some people have complicated narrowings and complete blockages which unfortunately are not suitable for PTCA. If you suffer from angina and many arteries are affected, a coronary bypass (see the question later on bypass surgery) may be the best option for you.

When my husband went into hospital for a PTCA, he had to sign a form saying he consented to having a stent inserted if it was found necessary during the operation. What is a stent and how does it work?

A stent is a metal mesh cage rather like a small meshwork tube (see Figure 3.6). It is made of thin flexible metal wire, and is fixed to a balloon with the balloon deflated. The original angioplasty balloon is removed – the wire is still in the artery so we have access to the narrowing – and the balloon with the stent on it is passed along the wire to the narrowing. The balloon inside the stent is inflated and the stent expands to the size of the balloon. It embeds itself into the artery wall and holds the artery open mechanically. The balloon is deflated and removed but the stent is permanently left behind. More than one stent may be used and the stent sizes vary according to the size of the arteries. Stents may be inserted without a prior balloon – this is known as direct stenting.

When will the cardiologist decide to insert a stent?

There are various reasons why the cardiologist decides to use a stent. The commonest are:

- if the angioplasty is not successful or the artery closes off;
- it is the cardiologist's choice (the most common reason);
- if the narrowing comes back 4–6 months after angioplasty;

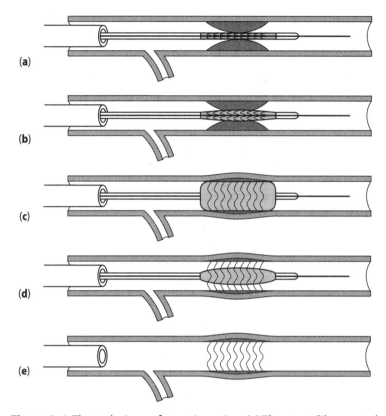

Figure 3.6 The technique of stent insertion. (**a**) The stent (like a metal cage) on balloon catheter is positioned at the problem site. (**b**) The balloon catheter is then inflated. (**c**) The stent is fully expanded and (**d**) left in place after the balloon has been deflated. (**e**) The stent remains expanded inside the artery.

- if the artery is large and the narrowing short, as the recurrence rate with a stent is reduced to 10–15%;
- if the narrowing is within a vein used for coronary bypass.

Stents are now used in over 90% of cases because of the better long-term results, with only 15% getting a narrowing within the stent after

6 months (this figure rises to 30% with the balloon on its own). If possible, they are placed directly without using a balloon beforehand as this reduces the risk of a complication.

Drug-eluting stents have been developed and are widely used because they have better than 95% long-term success. These have a drug coated on the metal stent, which acts to stop any further narrowing occurring. They are much more expensive than ordinary stents, which are now known as bare metal stents, but obviously reduce the chances of a repeat procedure. They may be particularly important in people with a higher risk of recurrence – those who have had a recurrence already, people with diabetes, and when the artery being stented is small.

I need an MRI scan. Do I tell the radiologist about my stents?

Yes. Routine MRI scanning is safe in all patients who have had a stent in place for 6 weeks. Stainless steel stents may displace in the first 6 weeks, but other makes remain secure. The chances of a stainless steel stent moving are minimal, however, so that MRI in an emergency should go ahead. Non-urgent cases should play safe and wait 6 weeks.

I was not offered a stent as a choice. Why was this?

This is most likely because angioplasty alone gave an excellent result. Stents are not as successful in smaller arteries, so this may have been the reason. Sometimes the arteries are too tortuous to allow a stent to pass through.

I am on tablets only at the moment for my angina. Is angioplasty or stenting better than medications?

Angioplasty or stenting can relieve any pain that medications have failed to control. They do not, however, provide any benefits compared to medication for preventing heart attacks. They are used only if conventional medical treatment does not give you relief from pain and a good quality of life. Angioplasty is a safe and effective procedure, but any operation has a slight risk, which you should avoid if possible.

I have been told that I need an angioplasty. I would prefer not to have an operation. Am I being overcautious?

Probably not. Because a narrowing looks suitable for a balloon, that doesn't mean that it is the best treatment. Angina from a narrowing in a branch vessel that is not a danger to life will usually settle with drug treatment, and the angioplasty option can be saved for later. As angioplasty in research studies has not been shown to improve (or shorten) life expectancy, it must be used selectively and it is then a very effective procedure. Using any procedure in every circumstance invites complications and devalues what is a useful form of therapy.

I am worried about having angioplasty done. Is there any chance that I will not get through the operation?

You have a greater than 99% chance of survival. These statistics include emergency operations and very sick people – routine cases like yours have a lower risk.

When will the doctor decide that I should have an angioplasty?

If you have angina and your tablets are not controlling it, the doctor will probably refer you for an angioplasty, if the narrowings are suitable. You will have an 80–90% chance of being relieved of your angina as a result.

I have just undergone an angioplasty with a stent and now been given some medication called clopidogrel. What is this drug for?

This is a powerful aspirin-like drug that prevents clotting on stents until they fully bed in. You usually start taking it about 6 hours before the procedure with a 'loading dose' of 300–600 mg. You will then take at least 75 mg daily for 4 weeks with a bare metal stent. Most doctors use it with aspirin also. Clopidogrel 75 mg daily is also used as an alternative in those unable to tolerate aspirin. Clopidogrel is also used in patients with unstable angina (see the earlier section *Symptoms*) as it reduces the complication rate. Skin rashes are the commonest side effect, and you may also notice that you bruise easily.

I have a drug-eluting stent in place and have been told to take clopidogrel and aspirin together for a year – is that correct?

Drug-eluting stents are vulnerable to clotting just like bare metal stents but they also have a late clotting risk when clopidogrel is stopped. Though this is not common it can be serious so doctors advise clopidogrel and aspirin for at least a year, and for some people, indefinitely. Clopidogrel has to be stopped for at least 5 days if you need an operation, such as a hernia repair, to avoid bleeding. A drug-eluting stent may therefore not be used if you plan to have non-heart surgery soon after the procedure.

Now that I have had an angioplasty, which has cured me of my angina pain, can I throw away all those tablets?

No, not all! You will need to continue with aspirin, cholesterol-lowering tablets and blood pressure tablets, if necessary. Any tablets that you take for angina might be reduced or stopped. Ask your doctor first – do not stop any medication without advice.

My wife has just come out of hospital where she underwent an angioplasty. She wasn't allowed to drive herself home. Why?

A week off is recommended. If you are recovering satisfactorily, you can then start driving again. The DVLA need not be notified but car insurance companies must be informed. For Group II driving, see the question below.

I hold a Group II licence and drive a lorry for a living. Will I lose my job and livelihood after angioplasty?

Driving is not recommended anyway if you have angina, even if your symptoms are controlled on medical treatment. This is a safety rule to protect the general public in case you should lose control of the vehicle during an attack. If you have heart failure (see Chapter 5), the DVLA can refuse you a licence. After a heart attack, bypass or angioplasty, you should stop professional driving for 6 weeks and you will only be allowed to resume if you have no symptoms and are able to complete an exercise test to the required standard.

How many people who have undergone angioplasties or stent insertion will have to then have an urgent bypass operation?

Only about 1 in 100.

My doctor mentioned a PCI – what is this?

PCI stands for *percutaneous coronary intervention* and this term covers both balloons and stents.

Bypass surgery

I have had medication and lots of tests for angina. I am now being offered bypass surgery. Why do I need this?

Operations for coronary artery disease are usually designed to improve the blood supply to the heart. A decision by the consultant as to whether to advise an operation for you is based on your case history and on several special tests, including an

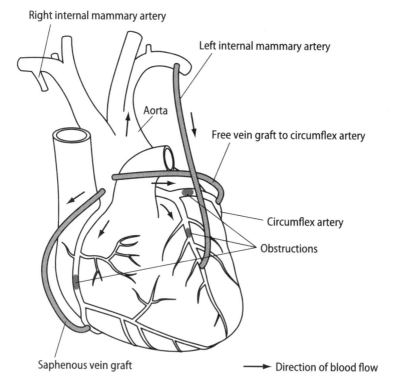

Figure 3.7 Diagram of coronary artery bypass surgery. Veins are used from the aorta to beyond the blockage and the mammary arteries taken directly from inside the chest.

electrocardiogram, an exercise test and an angiogram (see the section *Angiogram* earlier in this chapter). This last test is the most crucial one for bypass operations as it demonstrates the exact position and extent of the narrowings. An operation may be advised because of the severity of the symptoms or the extent of the disease or both. The operation may be performed to make you feel better, to prevent a heart attack or to correct life-shortening disease, thus giving you a longer and more active life.

Can you tell me what the bypass operation is all about?

The most common operation for angina is a coronary artery bypass. The full name is *coronary artery bypass graft* or CABG – often referred to as 'cabbage'.

A portion of vein is carefully removed from the leg and attached to the affected coronary artery beyond the narrowing. The other end of the vein is attached to the aorta, the main artery leading from the heart (see Chapter 1). In other words, the narrowing or obstruction is bypassed, just as a road bypass can avoid bottlenecks in towns. Several of these vein grafts may be placed, often one to each of the three major coronary artery branches. Frequently the graft is made with the left and right mammary artery from inside the chest (Figure 3.7). The radial artery is more frequently used now and taken from your lower arm between the wrist and elbow. Artery bypasses are believed to be stronger and longer lasting than vein bypasses. In each case your body can put up with the loss of the vein or artery used for the bypass.

In order to do these operations, the surgeon requires your heart to stop beating; so the heart and lungs are rested while the body is kept going by a heart-lung bypass machine. The operation is carried out through an incision down the front of the chest.

I read that some people can have a bypass without the need for a heart-lung machine – is this keyhole surgery?

Not really keyhole, but in selected cases the bypass can be done with the heart still beating. This is known as 'off-pump'. In appropriate cases the results are good and there may be fewer complications. The surgeon will decide who is suitable, based on the angiogram and medical history.

I am rather confused about the differences between the cardiologist and the surgeon – aren't they the same?

No. The cardiologist is a medical doctor and heart specialist who makes the diagnosis, investigates and treats you, and decides what is best to be done. The surgeon is a medical 'plumber' who puts in the bypasses and heart valves. When the job is done, the surgeon usually hands you back to the cardiologist to keep an eye on you. The cardiologist and surgeon work closely as a team to advise on and time the best treatment for you.

My doctor says that my heart has done its own bypass – what does he mean?

The coronary arteries link up through very small branches – they don't come to a full stop. This means that the left coronary artery can supply the right via the links, and vice versa. If these branches enlarge, they may fill a blocked artery backwards (see Figure 3.8). This means, for example, that a blocked right coronary artery may get its blood supply from the left system. The enlarging arteries are known as collaterals. Collaterals develop over time and can be encouraged by regular exercise. If you 'develop collaterals', so that a blocked artery gets its blood supply from another artery, it is then as if you have done your own bypass because, in effect, the blockage has been bypassed by your own arteries.

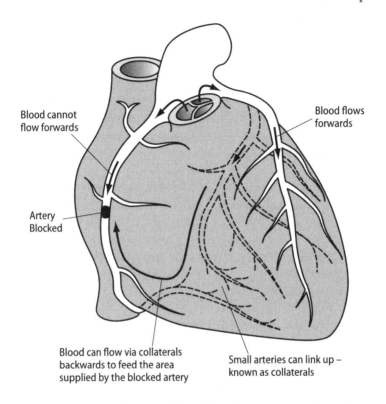

Blood cannot
flow forwards

Blood flows
forwards

Artery
Blocked

Blood can flow via collaterals
backwards to feed the area
supplied by the blocked artery

Small arteries can link up –
known as collaterals

Figure 3.8 Developing collaterals – doing your own bypass.

What do you use for a bypass operation if there are no suitable veins?

You have two arteries in the chest that can be used, two spare ones in the arms and also in the abdomen. The surgeon will find a way around the problem.

My doctor has recommended a bypass operation, but after all I've read about it, I don't think I want to have it done. Am I being used as a guinea pig?

The risks of severe coronary artery disease are higher if you do nothing. It is always important to discuss your own risks so that you and your family know where you stand. Risks will vary with age, how strong your heart muscle is and the extent of the coronary disease. On average, 98 patients in 100 pull through and two therefore do not. So you have a 98% rate of success but, if you are one of the other 2%, you have a 100% chance of dying. The odds are heavily on your side but it is important to understand what the statistics mean. If, for example, I told you that, because the operation is difficult, you had a 98% chance of living, you would feel differently to hearing that you had a one in 50 chance of dying, even though the figures mean exactly the same!

How long will a bypass graft last?

It used to be said that bypass surgery lasted 10 years, but these figures are out of date. The mammary artery bypass has a better than 90% chance of working for longer than 15 years after surgery. The veins can still harden and narrow but, with the use of aspirin and cholesterol-lowering medication, the length of time these bypasses last is improving all the time. The success depends on dealing with those factors that you have some control over, in particular high cholesterol levels, smoking and high blood pressure.

What happens before the bypass operation?

The surgeon who is going to perform the operation will examine you and explain what is planned. It is a great help for you to have your teeth checked by your own dentist well beforehand so that last-minute treatment can be avoided. This is to make sure there is no hidden infection that might affect the operation. Blood samples will be taken for tests; an electrocardiogram and a chest X-ray will also be taken. You will be visited by the physiotherapist and intensive care unit nursing staff to explain details of treatment to you. Before the operation, the anaesthetist will check on your lungs and ask about any allergies. The anaesthetist is a very important member of the team – your breathing will be controlled whilst the operation is being carried out.

Your chest and legs will be carefully shaved and you will be given a special antiseptic soap to clean the skin in several baths or showers. You will not have any food or drink for 4 hours before the anaesthetic is due. About 1 hour before the operation an injection will be given which will make you drowsy. The next thing you will know is waking up in the intensive care unit with the operation completed. The operation will take about 2–4 hours.

Why is the intensive care unit different to a normal ward?

The intensive care unit (ICU) is a halfway house between the operating theatre and the ward. You can be carefully observed there until you are again fit to be left to your own devices. Immediately after the operation you will still be fully anaesthetised and on a breathing machine. On awakening several hours later, you will have a tube in your mouth attached to the breathing machine, so that for a little while you will not be able to speak properly. This can be frightening at first and frustrating. However, as soon as you are fully awake, the tube is removed. As you are likely to be very thirsty at this time, you may take sips of water. The ICU is busy and noisy with lots of sophisticated machines. They are all there to help you and make sure the operation is a success. You may find it hard to rest. As soon as the nursing staff consider that it is safe to do so, you will be transferred to the main ward. You may feel that you have lost a day or are 'jet-lagged' and it is easy to be confused, but matters soon right themselves and you will soon feel yourself again.

One of the first visitors to the ICU is the physiotherapist. During the operation there is a tendency for your bronchial tubes to collect sputum and become blocked, causing small areas of collapse in the lungs. These then have to be fully expanded again by deep breathing and coughing with the encouragement and assistance of the physiotherapist. Naturally, after such an operation, your chest will be sore and you may be somewhat anxious about exerting yourself. However, with proper pain-killing injections and tablets, and knowing that there is no danger of 'bursting' stitches, you will soon overcome this fear. Giving up smoking as long as possible before the operation will greatly help in this respect.

What happens on the normal ward when I get transferred?

As far as operations go, bypass surgery is not one of the most painful, but many people often complain of feeling a bit low in spirits for a few days afterwards. This is only temporary and may be accompanied by other symptoms such as fatigue, poor concentration, slight blurring of vision, loss of taste, a disturbance of sleep pattern with drowsiness during the day, and restlessness and sweating at night. All these symptoms very rapidly pass off and are no cause for alarm. If it hurts to cough, clutch a small pillow to your chest (or better still a teddy bear – a present for your recovery!).

If you become constipated, mention it to the Ward Sister who will provide a mild laxative.

After one or two days, you will be encouraged to get out of bed and walk about. People vary greatly in their speed of recovery and getting up and about. There are no set rules – so if someone else appears to be doing better than you, it does not mean that anything is wrong. There is no competition involved! The nurses and physiotherapists will encourage you to get on your feet as fast as you can manage it without becoming exhausted.

You will usually be given support stockings for your legs, to prevent swelling and to keep your circulation moving. It is important that, when you are resting, you keep your legs raised on a stool or in bed, to avoid swelling during the first few days.

After about 6 to 7 days, any stitches will be removed from your chest and leg. You can have a bath if you want one. Leg wounds take longer than most to heal, and there may be a discharge of clear fluid, especially if your leg is not kept raised. This is not serious but should be pointed out to your doctor. It may feel a little numb just above the ankle on the inside of your leg.

Is it normal to get chest pains after the operation?

Muscular pains are common and can affect the chest, neck and back. They usually wear off over 2–3 weeks but can remind you of the operation for 2–3 months. Occasionally, bone and joint pain is a significant problem and anti-inflammatory tablets are prescribed. Most pains settle with simple painkillers, e.g. paracetamol or the stronger co-dydramol.

Can I lie on my side after a bypass operation?

You can lie in any position that you find comfortable.

Can the wound from a bypass operation fall apart?

No – your breastbone is wired together and you cannot undo the stitches or damage the operation. Very rarely the breastbone does not heal quickly and a click will be heard.

I am told that bypass surgery will make a large scar. Can't it be done by keyhole surgery?

Keyhole surgery is a media phrase – it does not happen in real life. In a few carefully selected cases, a bypass operation can be done without the need to open the breastbone or stop the heart. A cut is made to the side of the breastbone through three or four ribs and, whilst the heart is still beating, the surgeon constructs the bypass. Recovery is quicker than after a full bypass operation. It is a new procedure that is very appealing to the public, but applicable *only to a small number of people*, and it needs more testing to prove its effectiveness. If you are offered this option, ask about your particular surgeon's results and whether you will be entered in a research study to judge the success. Some surgeons are now opening only the lower end of the breastbone, which means that women can wear lower-cut garments, if they wish, without the scar showing.

> *I had a bypass some weeks ago. My scar is still tender. Why is this?*

At the end of the operation, wires are used to pull the breastbone together and hold it firm for healing – these are not usually removed. It sounds as though you are one of the small number of people who feel the ends of these wire stitches. This may settle down or only be an occasional problem; however, occasionally they can give trouble. The problem can usually be pinpointed by pressing with a finger. If this problem occurs, the wires can be removed under anaesthesia by your surgeon, because once the breastbone has healed the wires are no longer necessary.

> *My chest scar is pink and overgrown, following my bypass operation. Can it be improved?*

Occasionally, an operation scar may become pink and enlarges like a ridge. This is known as a *keloid*. It can be tender, itchy and unsightly. If it is a problem, steroid creams can be tried in order to relieve the discomfort. If it is intolerable, the scar can be cut out and then deep X-ray treatment given to stop the skin cells enlarging again.

> *I am due out of hospital in a few days after a successful bypass operation. What problems might I have?*

Most people go straight home providing there is someone there to help. If you live alone, it is best to spend the first 2 weeks with relatives or friends but, if this is not possible, your doctor should arrange, preferably before the operation, for your convalescence in a convalescent home. You will be given a supply of painkillers, a letter for your family doctor and advice on aspirin, diet and cholesterol medication. If you suffered from high blood pressure beforehand, this usually returns after the operation and will need careful checking. Almost certainly your blood pressure medications will need restarting.

When you return home, you may feel tired for a week or two. Although you are not exerting yourself, your body is doing a lot of repair work during this time.

How will I know that my bypass operation has been successful?

Your angina will be much less or non-existent. You will be less short of breath and have much more energy. You may say to yourself, 'I didn't realise how tired I had been', as you discover a new lease of life. A bypass should be a new start for you and your heart.

What exercise can I do on leaving hospital after my bypass operation?

Regarding exercise, you can do what you like within the bounds of commonsense! Unless carried to extremes, exercise will not hurt you. Any excess exercise will simply make you feel exhausted, and you can use this as a sign by which to pace yourself as you regain your fitness. In fact, regular exercise is an important factor in rehabilitation (see Chapter 10).

There is no reason to avoid normal sexual activities (see Chapter 8). The main problem may be pain from the muscles in the chest. If there are any problems do not avoid the subject, ask for help from your own doctor. Hairs on men's chests are prickly when they regrow and their partners may find this uncomfortable. A small soft pillow placed over the chest between partners can help.

I have a small garden at home. I'm due for a bypass operation next month. When will I be able to start gardening again?

Gardening is a good, rewarding form of exercise. Pace yourself doing the light work at first (weeding, dead-heading). Kneel down rather than bend over, to avoid muscular chest pain. Dig light soil but avoid any heavy clay soil until you are fully recovered. Cutting the grass should be possible after 3–4 weeks if the mower is light (such as a hover type). Avoid heavy work (lifting bags of fertiliser) or pushing a heavy roller mower until 6–8 weeks, when you should be back to normal.

I have been told that I should go on a cardiac rehabilitation programme. What does this involve and do I really need it, now that I feel so much better?

These programmes are strongly recommended as they give you structured advice on exercise and help you get out and about to meet others; these gatherings are a great boost to your confidence. In fact, you should positively demand to go on one! If one is not offered to you, make enquiries from the hospital where you had the operation or, if this a long distance away, ask your doctor or local cardiac unit. Rehabilitation programmes have been proved to help you get back to a normal life quicker, and there is now evidence that, if you follow all the advice, you will prevent problems in the future. You discover that you are not alone and you will find help is plentiful and advice freely given.

Are rehabilitation programmes just about exercise?

No – they offer lots of general advice. They assess whether you are anxious or depressed, advise on stress and how to relax, and you can raise any concerns you might have, for example, about resuming sexual activity, diet or which medication you need to take.

Now that I am back home after my bypass operation, how soon can I start driving again?

You should be able to drive your car 4 weeks after the operation. Check first with your doctor. The DVLA does not need to be notified but your car insurance company does. If you drive a heavy goods vehicle, you will have to pass an exercise test 6 weeks after the operation (see the section *Angioplasty*).

I would like to have a holiday now that I have had my bypass – would this be a good idea?

Yes indeed. A period of relaxation in a warm climate helps recovery. Airlines prefer you to wait 6 weeks before travelling and this is a good time in your recovery as it helps you get back to full strength. If an emergency arises and you need to travel by plane before the 6 weeks, there is usually no problem, but you may need a doctor's letter saying that it is all right to travel. Some travel insurance companies also require a letter. At the airport, the wires in your chest do not usually set off the alarms, but as the equipment's sensitivity varies from airport to airport, you may rarely set the alarm off. Stents do not usually sound the alarms either, but pacemakers do (see Chapter 6). After an angioplasty or stent placement, you may travel sooner – even within a week, although the doctor usually advises waiting 7–14 days.

How soon can I go back to work after a bypass operation?

If you were able to work before the operation, you should be back at work 2–3 months later. If your job involved hard physical labour or long working hours, ideally you should try to find a less strenuous job. However, hard physical work is safe if you become strong and fit again – ask the rehabilitation team to advise on strength-building exercises. If you are over 60 years of age, you should think about early retirement if this is financially possible.

I feel very tired with angina and I am looking forward to having my bypass operation. Will I really feel better after surgery?

You should feel fitter and stronger with much less or no angina. Many people feel much less fatigued.

I didn't really see the purpose of bypass surgery, but am prepared to undergo it if I can guarantee avoiding this terrible pain. I couldn't bear the thought of the operation not working. How can I stop my angina returning later?

Follow the guidelines on weight, exercise and cholesterol in Chapter 2.

- Do not smoke.

- Make sure your blood pressure is normal and your cholesterol low. Your target LDL cholesterol should be below below 2.0 if possible. Once you have achieved this, keep it down. The target is lower for those who have undergone bypass surgery (1.7–1.8) in order to protect the veins that have been used from narrowing and hardening.

- Take charge of yourself and make sure you have your life under control as much as possible.

- Do not sit back and let others look after you all the time.

How long will I be in hospital following bypass surgery?

A total of 7 to 8 days on average. Older people and more complex cases may be kept in a little longer.

OTHER TREATMENTS FOR ANGINA

Most other treatments for angina have no scientifically proven benefit. That said, many people with angina do better with attention and encouragement.

Complementary therapies which encourage relaxation may be useful if you are stressed. In the 1930s it was shown that even placebo (inactive) tablets could be helpful, relieving pain in a third of people with angina. Any effects with unproven treatment may therefore be the results of the placebo effect. As long as complementary treatment – be it herbs, acupuncture or reflexology – does no harm, feel free to try it. Bear in mind that, if the treatments were really proven to be useful, all doctors would be recommending them!

People who recommend these treatments tend to deride the scepticism sometimes shown by doctors but, even so, often do not provide the proof of success or submit the therapy to scientific validation. If someone could prove to me that massaging your right big toe was safe and relieved angina, I'd be the first to recommend it. I would have to advise you on the evidence (called evidence-based medicine) and there is none so far. Lots of people started using beta carotene for heart disease and cancer. Proper clinical trials have shown no benefit for this but did raise anxieties about adverse effects (see the section *Risks of high cholesterol levels* in Chapter 2). If you want to try an alternative approach, first be sure it is safe, then ask what proof there is. Always remember that isolated dramatic cases could be the result of the placebo factor.

I am not too sure what the 'placebo factor' means. Can you explain this to me?

Placebo translated from Latin means 'I will please'. A placebo effect is a benefit that cannot be explained by chemical actions from drugs or any scientific form of treatment. The benefit may be due to your belief (hope) that a treatment will work or just your total confidence in the doctor or alternative medicine practitioner ('This doctor is good; he will make me better'). Doctors use placebos to act as controls for their scientific preparations. Typically, they will test a new drug for angina and compare it with a placebo in such a way that neither you nor your doctor know which preparation is being taken. This is known as a 'double blind trial' and is a means of making sure that a new drug really does convey a benefit.

Could alternative medicine with acupuncture, homeopathy or herbal therapy just be a placebo effect?

You have put your finger on the problem! Alternative therapies have not undergone the rigorous testing that doctors would like to see. However, it is difficult to study alternative therapies as there is little motivation from large drug companies to fund such studies, since herbs cannot be patented. Alternative medicine practitioners believe there is no need for this sort of study, as they feel the ideas have been practised for many years.

What types of alternative therapy are available for people with heart problems?

Acupuncture uses needles at various points of the body to release energy (*chi*) and this is believed to be essential to good health. *Homeopathy* uses minute quantities of substances which produce similar symptoms to those experienced by people with heart problems, in the belief that resistance will develop. *Herbalism* uses plant-based preparations (often in an alcohol base) believed to restore good health. Herbal medicine is known as phytotherapy (plant therapy) and is quite separate from homeopathy.

I have heard that herbs can be helpful in heart disease and
angina. Can you give me some advice?

Any alternative therapy (such as herbs) should not replace an accurate conventional diagnosis but only be tried once the diagnosis has been made and the safety of that treatment established. Some of the effects that have been claimed for herbs and other plants include:

- breakdown of plaques in arteries (alfalfa, garlic, hawthorn, mistletoe);

- relaxation (lemon balm, lily-of-the-valley, St John's wort, valerian);

- relief of anginal symptoms (pineapple);

- lowering of hypertension (bugle, hawthorn, mistletoe, skullcap, yarrow);

- relief of stress and anxiety (camomile, skullcap, St John's wort);

- circulation stimulation (cayenne, ginger, hawthorn);

- diuretic (dandelion, lily-of-the-valley, yarrow);

- antioxidant (garlic);

- lowering of cholesterol (ginger, motherwort, onion);

- reduction of clotting (gingko, onion);

- relief of palpitations (motherwort).

None of the claims for these herbs has reliably passed scientific scrutiny, yet a whole industry exists based on the assertions made. Only garlic has been studied in any depth and, whilst there seems to be some benefit, it should be considered a supplement not an alternative (see the question on garlic in Chapter 9). In other words, don't stop your medication, which has been scientifically proved to help, but do try complementary treatments that can be bought in reputable chemists' shops if you want to, following the advice on the information leaflets.

You keep emphasising the importance of going to reputable shops to buy herbal medicine. Isn't all the information we need on the label?

Not necessarily! A recent study looked at 30 different boxes of feverfew, used to help migraine and arthritis. Only two preparations contained any feverfew at all. The problem is that medications are rigorously checked but herb preparations are not (currently) regulated. Drugs on the Internet are totally uncontrolled.

Are Chinese herbs the same as our herbal medicines and can they help?

Chinese herbal medicine is based on a different philosophy and uses different preparations and diagnostic techniques to those in the West, so it is considered a separate branch of herbal medicine. Again, many claims are made, but there is little scientific evidence available. When I studied one Chinese herb recommended for angina, compared to placebo all it did was to cause more headaches!

Are you in favour or against alternative methods of treatment?

If any treatment makes you feel better and does no harm, I cannot be against it. You must, however, have a full medical history and examination to make sure that nothing is being missed. Herbal medicine is slow-acting and best for chronic conditions, so it may help angina. Certain herbs in excess can lead to side effects – parsley in very large quantities can cause liver damage, celery and angelica can cause the skin to be sensitive to sunlight, and many other herbs can cause stomach upsets. Some are even poisonous! This means that you should go only to a qualified medical herbalist who knows how to handle the herbs and select the right ones for you. The same goes for homeopathy and acupuncture – only go to accredited people. There are some addresses in Appendix 2.

I thought alternative medicine practitioners were all trained. Isn't this so?

No. Anyone can set up as a specialist in complementary or alternative medicine and there are no government requirements for training. This means that in the wrong hands, you could be harmed or have a medical condition missed. Always check if the practitioner is registered, has qualifications, is insured and is well established in practice in the area. Do not use the Internet unless it is a reputable pharmacy.

Why are doctors so sceptical about alternative medicine?

Doctors, and for that matter nurses and other trained medical people, have to qualify to certain standards and practise their craft following strict guidelines and codes of ethics. They are naturally suspicious of those who do not have to follow these rigorous rules and can make claims which are not or cannot be scientifically proven. Doctors are now being urged to practise only 'evidence-based medicine' which is medicine absolutely proven to be of benefit. They obviously wonder why others are not strictly policed.

Do you think there is place then for alternative medicine or should I ignore it?

Yes there is a place for alternative medicine, provided that a full medical assessment has been performed on you and that the practitioner is fully qualified. Quality of life can be improved by many things, including a placebo. Provided that there is no evidence of harm, alternative treatments can be tried. There is no evidence that alternative medicine will lengthen your life, so if your life is threatened by heart disease, conventional medicine will be essential for your protection.

Can complementary therapies do any harm?

The short answer is yes – so always go to your doctor if you are taking these products; if you have a heart condition, check before you try them. Here are some reported dangers.

- Ma huang (Ephedra) used for weight loss and energy enhancement may cause stroke, heart attacks and sudden death.

- Chelation has killed some patients.

- Siberian ginseng can falsely elevate digoxin drug levels, leading to incorrect decisions.

- Gingko inhibits clotting and may increase the effect of warfarin (ginger, garlic and ginseng do this also).

- St John's wort and gingko can deepen the effects of anaesthetics, cause blood pressure problems and bleeding. St John's wort can cause a fatal irregularity of the heartbeat – avoid it!

I have read in the paper about laser surgery. This sounds exciting – is it being used everywhere?

The word 'laser' sells newspapers and excites the reader. Laser balloons have come and gone because of a lack of benefit. The technique of transmyocardial laser revascularisation (doctors like long names!) is a treatment using lasers to create tiny channels in the heart muscle from the inside. It can be done by opening the chest (surgically) or via the arteries, like a catheter procedure. Patients for whom angioplasty or bypass surgery are not suitable can undergo this procedure, the idea being that blood from the inside of the ventricle (pump) feeds the muscle via the channels. The results vary a lot and it is still experimental. So, if this procedure is offered to you, make sure that there are no other options (if need be, get a second opinion), and that the centre has ethical approval and a lot of experience. (There are cowboy doctors as well as cowboy builders!)

What drugs should I be on to help stop my angina problems coming back?

All patients with coronary disease should be taking:

- aspirin (or clopidogrel);
- a statin (dose increased to get LDL 2.0 mmol/litre or less);
- a beta-blocker (such as bisoprolol 2.5–5 mg or atenolol 50 mg daily); and
- an ACE inhibitor (such as perindopril up to 8 mg, ramipril 5–10 mg daily) or an AII inhibitor (such as valsartan, candesartan, losartan, irbesartan) providing there are no specific contraindications or side effects.

If you are not on one of these drugs, ask why.

Drugs are much cheaper on the Internet – is it safe to buy them?

If you buy drugs this way you have no idea what you are taking. There is no control over the content of the tablets, or of the 'vehicle' which is used to keep the drug in the tablet, which may be a banned substance. In addition, the content may clash with your prescribed drugs. So only buy from a reputable online pharmacy and not 'Dave' who can sell you Viagra for 50p a tablet.

4 | Heart attacks

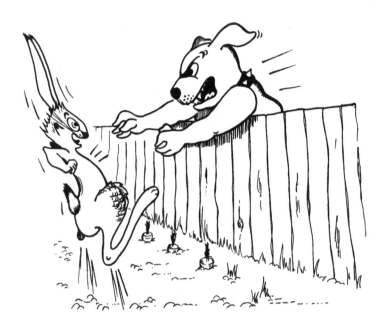

The medical term for a heart attack is *myocardial infarction* (pronounced 'myo-car-dee-al in-fark-shun'). The heart muscle is the myocardium; infarct means death – thus, death of heart muscle. Some people also use the term 'coronary' because the cause is a block of a coronary artery.

Every 30 seconds someone dies from coronary artery disease. It is the single most important cause of death for men and women. Coronary artery disease kills more people than all the cancers put together.

Will I be able to avoid a heart attack?

There is no guarantee (never say never!) but your risks can be lessened by heeding the following advice.

- Do not smoke (not one cigarette, not at all).

- Avoid passive smoking (sit in non-smoking areas; if your family smokes, send them outside to do so).

- Watch your blood pressure (know your reading).

- Know your cholesterol level and keep it low by diet, and medication if necessary (this is very important).

- Eat plenty of fresh fruit and vegetables.

- Keep your weight down and take plenty of exercise.

- Enjoy alcohol in moderation.

Just as you service your car – service your body.

Can you tell me what causes a heart attack?

A heart attack occurs when an area of heart muscle is deprived of blood because of a blockage in a coronary artery. As the muscle no longer has oxygen to feed it, it begins to die, chemicals build up and pain is felt. The cause is usually a clot forming on an area of narrowing in an artery (see Chapter 2).

I have recently heard that heart attacks can be caused by exhaust pollution. Is this true?

Recently, a statistical link has been reported between car exhaust pollution and heart attacks, with those most at risk being pedestrians, cyclists and drivers. Links like this have been shown before (for example, in railwaymen in fume-filled tunnels) but no medical proof exists that it causes a heart attack, and there could be other interpretations of the association. An association does not mean a cause, and most links like this raise more questions than are resolved. It is of course interesting, but there is little we can do about it other than change our travel methods on a large scale.

SYMPTOMS

What are the symptoms of a heart attack?

A lmost always there is chest pain. It usually builds up to become severe. It lasts longer than half an hour and, unless treated,

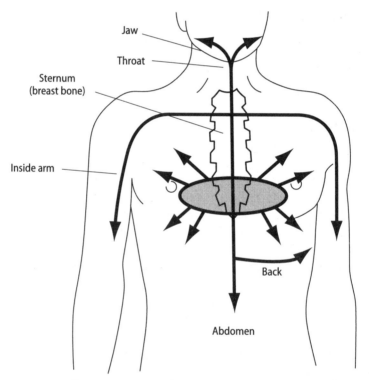

Figure 4.1 Site and radiation of heart pain.

may go on for 4–6 hours or more. The pain is most often across your chest and feels like a weight or a tightness. Some people describe it with a clenched fist as if the pressure or squeezing of the pain resembles the clenching of the fist. The pain is rarely sharp like a knife and cannot be pointed to by one finger as it is spread across the chest. The pain comes from the same place, even if you change your position from standing to sitting or lying down (see Figure 4.1).

You may also get pain down your arms, usually the inside, to your wrists. The left arm is more often affected than the right. It can go to your jaw, throat, back or stomach. The pain may be severe, causing sweating, and be associated with feeling sick (nausea) or vomiting. So, get help fast if you have:

- a heavy feeling – a feeling like a weight or pressure, or a squeezing feeling like a band in the chest – that lasts longer than 20 minutes and builds up (heart attack pain usually builds up rather than being at its worst when it starts);

- pain from your chest, going to your neck, jaw or arms (left more common than right) and lasting longer than 20 minutes;

- pain (or discomfort) along with nausea, sweating, feeling faint or short of breath.

Are there any warning signs that might point to an impending heart attack?

Many people complain of 'indigestion' for some days or weeks beforehand. What they have been experiencing is angina.
It is quite common for people who have had a heart attack to say that they have been very tired in the previous 3–6 months. Some complain of breathlessness (the tightness across the chest has a breathless feeling about it) and dropping off to sleep watching TV. Others have noticed an increased tendency to snore and irritability: feeling 'out of sorts', 'just not themselves'.

A new warning sign is that of men complaining of difficulty getting an erection. The blood vessels to the penis do not function properly and can reflect problems with the blood vessels to the heart. Erection problems in men are caused by smoking, raised cholesterol, blood pressure or diabetes – exactly the same as for the coronary arteries! Play safe and go to the doctor. If you are worried about a friend or relative, do not take no for an answer – get them to see a doctor. If you think it is a heart attack, do not delay: for every 1 hour's delay, one life in every hundred will be lost – dial the emergency services (999 in the UK).

I know that I get angina and have learnt to recognise the symptoms. How will I recognise the difference between the pain of angina and that of a heart attack?

Angina is the result of a temporary shortage of oxygen available to the heart muscle and is usually caused by exercise (such as walking up a hill) or strong emotion, especially anger (see Chapter 3). The pain is most often a tightness or a weight on your chest that may spread to your neck or arms. Anginal pain passes off when you stop or reduce exercise or when you take a nitrate tablet or spray. It does not last longer than half an hour.

The cause of angina is narrowing of the coronary arteries. Think of the artery as a three-lane motorway and angina as the result of two lanes being coned off. All the traffic will get through if people travel slow enough but, at high speeds, three lanes will only go into one if someone stops to give way. If no one gives way there will be a crash blocking the third lane. This is what happens in a heart attack. A clot forms on the narrowed part to block the artery totally. Narrow coronary arteries are often described as being hardened or furred-up.

My brother has had a heart attack – according to the hospital. He says that he did not feel it happening. I thought a heart attack was painful.

Some heart attacks can be so minor that they are barely noticed, but others can be more severe. The severity depends on which part of the artery is affected. If you look at the diagram of the heart in Chapter 1 (Figure 1.1), you will see that there are two main arteries shown – the right and left. The left divides into two main trunks. These branch again and again into smaller branches or tubes (vessels), supplying blood to all of the heart muscle. A blockage in one of the tiny vessels means that only a very small part of the heart is deprived of blood. A blockage in a larger branch affects a much larger area of heart muscle. Because the blood can no longer get through and feed the heart and remove waste from the muscle, chemicals build up to produce pain, as if the heart had been bruised.

HEART ATTACK – THE EVENT

My mother has been told that she is 'at high risk' of a heart attack. I am her carer and am worried about her. What should I do if I think she is having a heart attack?

Your mother should rest completely in a comfortable position, preferably lying flat with her feet slightly raised. Make her avoid any exertion: if you are at home, the floor is best, not the bed if stairs are involved. Call the ambulance immediately (dial 999) and tell them that you think that your mother is having a heart attack. Make sure that you stay on the line long enough to tell them precisely where she is. If you know her doctor's name, contact the surgery immediately: the doctor may be able to start treatment before the ambulance arrives. If your mother has been given glyceryl trinitrate tablets or sprays for angina, then one or two tablets or sprays should be given. She should also chew 300 mg aspirin, or dissolve and swallow it, unless she is allergic to it or she has a recently (inside 1 month) proven stomach ulcer; if in doubt, give it anyway – the benefit is greater than the risk.

Why do we have to say 'heart attack' when calling an ambulance?

Some areas have specially equipped ambulances which can give immediate care to coronary patients – these are known as 'coronary ambulances'. The staff – often paramedics – are coronary trained and can deal with the situation and its problems with a great deal of expertise and skill.

We live in the country and fortunately have a very good local hospital. However, it does not have a coronary care unit like the general hospital 40 minutes away. Our doctor has advised us to go to the coronary care unit in the event of my husband having a heart attack. Why?

In the early hours after a heart attack, the build-up of chemicals can irritate the heart and upset the electrical system that controls the heartbeat. A very irregular rhythm known as *ventricular fibrillation* (VF) can occur. In effect, it is as if the heart has stopped; all that is happening is that the heart muscle (ventricle) is chaotically wriggling like a bag of worms (fibrillating), and there is no blood leaving the heart as a result. This can be corrected by prompt medical treatment so that normal heartbeats can be restored. Prompt treatment means being in the hands of the experts in a coronary care unit who can keep an eye on your husband hour by hour until the risk settles, usually after 24 hours.

Coronary care units employ highly trained nurses who deal with pain, monitor the heart and supervise specific treatments designed to minimise complications and speed recovery.

My partner is very stubborn and simply refuses to go to hospital.
He is getting on now and not strong. He has been a life-long
smoker. I do not want to upset him by making him go to hospital
if he had a heart attack. Would he be able to stay at home?

Some doctors believe it is safe for people to stay at home provided that suitable facilities and care are available. The danger period is usually within the first 12 hours; if this time has passed already and there are no problems, it is probably as safe to be at home. Older people like your partner may be happier at home also. Home care involves the family, district nurses and family doctor, and its quality will depend on their availability and workload.

It is unwise to be at home alone following a heart attack. If the heart attack has just happened, it is better to be in hospital, where everything is immediately to hand. This applies to young and old people of both sexes. There is clear evidence that otherwise fit people in their eighties benefit from thrombolysis (clot buster medication) and angioplasty (balloon treatment) where needed – and that means going to hospital.

Going to hospital

My husband has heart problems and I am told that he is 'at risk'.
If he had a heart attack, what actually happens after hospital
admission?

If your husband has a heart attack at home, an assessment is usually made in the ambulance. He will then go to the hospital casualty department; some hospitals have a 'fast-track' system and he would go straight to the Coronary Care Unit (CCU) or for an angiogram.

The hospital doctor will take blood to look for evidence of damage (enzymes). Contents of the muscle cells leak out when there is damage. They help the doctor determine the size of the attack. Routinely now, another chemical test for troponin is performed; this is very sensitive at identifying damage – doctors talk of 'trop positive' (damage) or 'trop negative' (no damage). A recording of the electrical activity of your husband's heart (ECG or EKG, see Chapter 3) will be taken at least once and will usually confirm the diagnosis and help identify the precise area of damage. Eight out of 10 heart attacks show on the first ECG and it is after this that clot buster drugs or angioplasty are offered. A chest X-ray will be taken to see if there is any fluid in his lungs.

Your husband will probably be given medication (morphine) to relieve pain and limit complications. Tablets or injections may be used to reduce fluid in his lungs (diuretics) and stabilise his heartbeats if there is any irregularity causing concern.

There are three sorts of medications which are most often used (unless there are specific reasons why they should not be given) because they protect the heart, improve survival and reduce complications (see the section *Treatment* in Chapter 3).

- Aspirin thins the blood to help prevent further clots. He will be able to take this in the soluble form, 75 mg/day, and will probably take it for the rest of his life.

- Beta-blockers are medications that slow the heart down and reduce blood pressure. They protect the heart from too much physical and mental stress. Because these medications can improve your husband's chances of survival after a heart attack, they will be probably be given long term. Commonly used preparations are atenolol, bisoprolol, propranolol, metoprolol and timolol.

- Angiotensin-converting enzyme inhibitors or ACE inhibitors help some people survive. Fewer people on these medications have heart failure and they help reduce the heart's tendency to enlarge after a heart attack. Commonly used tablets are captopril, lisinopril, enalapril, ramipril and perindopril.

In the coronary care unit (CCU), rest is crucial to allow his heart to recover. Visiting by immediate family only should be brief as he will often tire easily. Young children can often be upset by the visit so care is needed if they come to see him. A brief visit to see that 'daddy' or 'mummy' is okay may benefit both child and parent, but the child must be fully prepared for the sight of the equipment, which can be daunting. It may be better if a nurse takes the child into the unit in a matter of fact way; this can reduce the natural tendency for the family to become emotional at a time of great stress.

In the CCU meals are light, as heavy meals can increase the heart's work by 20%, and rest is really what is needed. Your husband will find fluids, soups and salads are the easiest options.

As part of life in the CCU, there are routine ECGs, chest X-rays and blood tests, all designed to monitor his progress.

My husband went straight for an angioplasty even in his outdoor clothes – why did they rush?

The paramedics or casualty staff will have diagnosed the heart attack and the best chance of saving the heart muscle from damage is to open the blocked artery as quickly as possible. This is known as a primary angioplasty and represents the state-of-the-art management. Time is of the essence so speed saves lives.

My husband has gone into a Coronary Care Unit. What will happen when he returns to the general ward?

Most people leave coronary care after 24–48 hours. Everyone is an individual, not a statistic, so some leave sooner than others. Once your husband is back on the cardiac or general ward, a restful atmosphere is still essential and visitors should be restricted to avoid fatigue. Fear and ignorance are the biggest problems at this stage, so it is very important for him to fully understand what is going on. Questions need answers, so do not suffer in silence worrying about something. The key to your husband's recovery will be for him and his family to participate actively in the rehabilitation process. Do not keep any facts from his family and friends, as this leads to emotional charades at a time when maximum support is needed.

He will normally leave hospital after 7–10 days, but your husband may be kept in a little longer if his doctor thinks that he needs longer to recover. During the recovery period he will be encouraged to increase his exercise gradually, and he will be given advice on how to live and eat healthily.

Just before discharge from hospital, or within 6 weeks of a heart attack, an exercise ECG on a treadmill will be arranged for him. This is designed to rule out any further heart trouble and allows the doctor and your husband to judge how well his recovery is progressing.

What drugs should a heart attack patient be taking on leaving hospital?

Drugs may be used to protect from further events and these are:

- aspirin or clopidogrel, or both;
- statins;
- beta-blockers;
- ACE inhibitors or AII antagonists.

He should also be taking written information explaining what has happened and what to do next. An appointment with cardiac rehabilitation is strongly recommended. Specific drugs may be used to control symptoms, such as diuretics (water tablets) to relieve fluid retention and breathlessness. All heart attack patients should understand what the medication is for – if unsure, always ask.

RECOVERY PERIOD

I always thought that having a heart attack was the end of the story. Now you give me the good news that nearly everyone recovers nowadays. Is this true?

The short answer is not everybody recovers, but the good news is that most people do. Indeed most people make a complete recovery and only a small number are left with a disabling limitation, such as chest pain on effort (angina) or excessive breathlessness. We can help most people get back on their feet, but sadly a small number, less than one in 10 cases, have suffered too much damage even for all the modern technology to overcome.

A friend of mine had a heart attack recently and is still in hospital. She rang me to say that she was coming out soon. Will she be completely dependent and unable to look after herself? What can she do for herself after leaving hospital?

Don't panic! The danger period has passed but, of course, going home means a change of environment with no friendly nurses immediately to hand to provide security and reassurance. Not surprisingly, I expect that she will feel uncertain, anxious and depressed for a while.

It is important for her not to be alone for the first 2 weeks after discharge from hospital so, if she normally lives alone, it is best for her to stay with relatives or friends who can provide the necessary support and, of course, be there to talk to. The hospital should have ensured that her doctor knows she is coming home so that a visit can be arranged by either the family doctor or practice nurse, to see how she is getting on. This may be worth confirming with the doctor's surgery. Special cardiac liaison nurses do home visits in some localities, providing an important link between patient and their family, family doctor and hospital.

I had a heart attack over a month ago and I now feel completely better. I am frustrated that my doctor wants me to vegetate at home! When will I be allowed to lead a normal life again after my heart attack?

Most people are back to normal 6–8 weeks after a heart attack and back at work within 2–3 months. Some people take early retirement because a favourable financial package has been offered, and they are getting close to retirement age anyway. This makes good sense. Women who were working part-time are less likely to go back, as their work was invariably an additional job to their other commitments. Career women, however, can get back to work as successfully as men do: of those who want to work, 80–90% will do so. If your heart was badly damaged, your doctor may advise you not to work, and you will also need to take into account how demanding your job was.

If you do go back to work, make sure that you maintain a healthy lifestyle with plenty of exercise, an active social and leisure life, and a good night's sleep to help recharge your batteries.

What should I do to help my recovery after my heart attack?

There are several important aspects to helping the recovery and these include:

- making sure that you take your medication, understanding why you have been given it, and taking it in the correct dose;

- losing weight if you need to;

- enjoying plenty of fresh fruit and vegetables;

- increasing physical activity sensibly;

- learning to relax and getting a good night's sleep; and

- avoiding cigarette smoking (active or passive).

I am on the mend after a heart attack – a nasty shock! How will I feel in myself when I return home?

After a heart attack it is common for both you and your family and friends to worry and be a bit fearful. The fears most people have are that:

- they might die;

- they will lose their sex life;

- they might have to give up work;

- they might have a physical disability.

They might also feel:

- angry about why it happened;

- guilty about not taking advice; and

- depressed that life, as you have known it, is finished and somehow you will be less of a person.

These feelings and fears are discussed more fully below. Most of them pass quickly as you make progress and recover, but it is always good to express any anxieties and worries to the hospital staff or your family doctor when you are home, because they can nearly always be explained and this will help you to overcome them.

Joining a rehabilitation programme is a very important means of coming to terms with what has happened and helping you to be positive about the future. Your spouse or partner is welcome to attend and the education, understanding and support provided soon restore your confidence, enabling you to return to a normal sex life and work.

Am I likely to get more chest pain after I have recovered from my heart attack?

Most people do not, but just a few do get angina. An exercise test will be organised for you and treatment arranged (see Chapter 3). Always tell your doctor if you get any pain. You don't have to put up with it – there are lots of things that your doctor will be able to do for you.

I am home from hospital after having had a heart attack. Will I need surgery or angioplasty in the future?

The first priority is to let your heart heal up. An exercise test may suggest that you have further problems and, if so, an angiogram will be arranged for you (see the section *Tests* in Chapter 3). If you have serious further trouble, you may be advised to have surgery or angioplasty so that these problems do not get worse. It is better to prevent further heart attacks by changing your lifestyle and taking the right medicine and treatment.

EMOTIONAL PROBLEMS AFTER A HEART ATTACK

Will I be able to resume a normal sex life after a heart attack?

The answer is definitely yes! Questions about sexual and emotional problems are asked by anyone who has had any serious health upsets, not just people with heart problems. This is such an important issue that it is covered in more detail in Chapter 8.

Why do I feel so angry about what has happened to me?

'Why did this happen to me?' and 'Why now?' are common questions asked. Heart attacks can occur at any time, not at a convenient time; they are always inconvenient. If you feel angry and bitter about what has happened, you are likely to be short of patience and irritable. You may take these feelings out on close friends and family; this is understandable but they too will be suffering. Remember that being angry is a stage in your recovery process and it will pass. Sometimes it is a good idea to discuss these feelings with someone who is not so close to you as family – that is why it is such a good idea to join a cardiac rehabilitation programme.

I still feel very moody at times after my heart attack. Why is this?

You may feel up and down, day by day, as you come to terms with what has happened. Don't worry about these mood swings or feeling as if you have 'the blues' – focus on resting and being positive about the future. Don't bottle your feelings up – talk to someone close, your family doctor or practice nurse. These feelings are all quite normal.

I am the one who has had a heart attack, but I now feel fine, perhaps a bit low sometimes; but my children really blame themselves over what happened. Why do they feel guilty?

Your family has been through a traumatic time also – they have been afraid of losing you and have had to put a brave face on every day. Children often feel guilty – teenagers in particular – that in some way they may have caused your heart attack. Explain to them that, although the heart attack was sudden (they all are), what caused it took years to develop and they could not be to blame. Talk a lot, don't suffer in silence or let your family suffer in silence. As the Americans say, 'let it all hang out' or these bad feelings will fester and become destructive.

I'm really depressed after my heart attack, which is unusual for me as I am usually 'bubbly'. My doctor tells me that this is normal after a heart attack. How will I know if I am 'medically' depressed rather than just 'down'?

Being down in the dumps at times is common for 2–3 months after a heart attack but this will lessen as you get back to normal. Some people may have been inclined to be depressed before a heart attack, and this can develop into a more significant medical problem. Constant irritability and heavy drinking are early signs. Other problems include:

- difficulty in sleeping;

- lack of energy;

- poor appetite;

- loss of interest in your old activities ('I can't be bothered to go visiting');

- unable to concentrate ('I pick up the paper, put it down, pick it up, forget what I have just read');

- paying less attention to your appearance.

More serious cases are associated with a feeling of no value, being worthless and having thoughts of suicide.

You must make sure that your doctor is aware of these feelings, as medication or counselling can help the way you feel. There is no need to put up with feeling depressed, nor for you and your family to suffer. If life seems desperate, phone the Samaritans or go to the hospital – seek help.

TREATMENT

What treatment will I be given when I leave hospital following my heart attack?

Some medication is prescribed as a matter of course because you will have a better chance of survival and complications can be prevented. Medication includes aspirin, clopidogrel, statins, beta-blockers and ACE inhibitors (see the section *Treatment* in Chapter 3). Not all medicines suit everyone and not everyone needs them, but you should be aware if you are taking them and, if not, why not. For some reason, not all people are given the medication that they need: only one-third of those people who should be on beta-blockers are prescribed them. Because you have a 25% better chance of survival if you are given beta-blockers, it is important to know why you haven't been given them. Ask you doctor why are you are not on them if you have not been prescribed these tablets.

Other tablets may be prescribed for specific problems, for example water pills (diuretics) to reduce fluid retention and help breathing, and special medication to regulate your heart rhythm if it has been upset by the heart attack.

Just as it is vitally important to know what you are being treated with, it is equally important not to discontinue any treatment without checking with the doctor first. Simply stopping medication is a dangerous policy, as you could suddenly get a rebound effect and risk another heart attack occurring. If you have side effects, tell your doctor so that your medication can be changed to another type.

If you had a heart attack whilst taking medication for another condition, such as high blood pressure or high cholesterol, it is essential to check whether treatments for these are still needed – they usually will be.

My husband has angina and I am worried that he may not survive a heart attack. What can I do if he has one suddenly – and what should I tell his friends to do?

Quick action is needed by you or his friends, as the muscle will stop working permanently if left without oxygen for 6 hours. The quicker you act, the better the chances of survival: getting help within 1 hour is better than within 2. He will have the very best chances of survival if you get help within the first 4 hours following the start of pain.

There are medications that can be used to break down the clot and open up the artery again. These are known as 'clot buster drugs' and the medical term for breaking down the clot is *thrombolysis* (pronounced 'throm-bo-lie-siss'). Aspirin helps break down clots as do streptokinase or tissue plasminogen activators (TPAs). As these medications thin the blood, they are not used when there is a risk of bleeding elsewhere, for example if someone has a stomach ulcer or has recently had surgery. If you think your husband has had a heart attack, and he is able, get him to crunch a 300 mg aspirin into small pieces and swallow it before the trip to hospital. Some pieces will be absorbed quickly through the lining of the mouth.

Clot buster drugs slightly increase the chances of a stroke, but this is offset by a major reduction (40%) in his chances of death from a heart attack. Streptokinase is less expensive than TPA, but TPA is more effective within 4 hours of a heart attack and the more frequently used. If he is given streptokinase, his body becomes sensitive to its effects, so it cannot be used again for at least 12 months, but TPA can be used as many times as is needed. People treated with these medications are given a card to carry with them for future reference.

Clot busters are not always successful but do work for 7 out of 10 people with heart attacks.

Is there an alternative to 'clot buster' drugs for heart attacks?

Apart from letting nature take its course, percutaneous trans-luminal coronary angioplasty (PTCA) is the only alternative. This is a means of unblocking arteries with a balloon and squashing the narrowings out of the way (see the section *Angioplasty* in Chapter 3 with Figure 3.5). PTCA can be performed if clot busters fail or the pain returns after the clot busters have been tried, if there is a reason why such medications cannot be used safely, or if you are admitted to a unit where angioplasty is routinely available. Angioplasty with a stent inserted is the most successful way of opening the blocked artery and limiting heart muscle damage and is now advocated as the preferred treatment if available (day or night).

We were so grateful that my brother did not die from his heart attack. Why do some but not others die from a heart attack?

Sometimes the attack is just too big for all the modern treatment to cope with, sometimes the treatment just doesn't work and some-times it's left too late. No matter how clever we are, there is always going to be a bad luck factor. However, advances have increased the chances of surviving from 76 to 93% over the last 10 years.

HELPING YOURSELF

Exercise

I have always hated exercise. Now that I have had a heart attack, and presumably should take things easy, my doctor tells me that I need to take more exercise. What exercise should I be doing?

Many people like you who have had a heart attack were not physically fit before their heart attack: perhaps, because of pressures of work, there was little time for sport or leisure activities. Exercise is very good for you, but it does need to be enjoyed rather than seen or felt as a punishment. Dynamic exercise, involving movement, e.g. walking, swimming, cycling, jogging, tennis, dancing and golf, is the most helpful. Isometric exercise, e.g. weight-lifting or press-ups, is not beneficial and should be avoided. Exercise should be undertaken every day but it is not compulsory, so avoid wet, cold and windy weather – consider walking in a new enclosed shopping mall if you have one near you. An exercise bicycle is a way of keeping up exercise when the weather is bad, and boredom can be avoided by putting the bike in front of the TV set.

Walking is very good exercise and it is cheap and safe. There is no need to take up jogging, if you don't want to – just walk briskly, climb stairs and avoid lifts if you can. Swimming is also good for the heart. At first, always stay in your own depth and do not dive in. Gradually increase to swimming some lengths of the pool as slowly as you like, and then speeding up.

Exercise should be increased gradually as the weeks go by. Some people feel unable to do much at first, and may even be afraid of doing anything at all or going out alone. Going out with relatives or friends helps but joining a rehabilitation programme, if possible, is the best way of regaining confidence and getting the maximum benefit.

During your first 2 weeks at home, do slightly more exercise each day in terms of distance and time. There is no need to be afraid of going up stairs or going for a walk. A useful plan is to cancel the daily paper and walk to the newsagent to collect it. This is exercise with a purpose: you can stop for a chat, and you know how long it takes to walk the distance to the shop, so the time it takes can be reduced as you speed up and get fitter.

It is a good idea to chart your exercise and how you are doing over the weeks following your heart attack. You may be surprised at how much you can already do and how much improvement you are making. Aim to walk briskly for 30–40 minutes at least five times a week and for over an hour if you need to lose weight. You can break this up, for example into two 20-minute walks.

By 6 weeks after your heart attack, you should be back to normal activity, or even better, because most people do not exercise enough normally. There is more information in Chapter 10.

How I should begin my exercises?

It is always important to warm up first. Do some bending and stretching, and then set off at a gradual pace, gently speeding up. At the end of the exercise, allow time to cool down. See Chapter 10 for more information.

You hear horror stories about the dangers of exercise, from slipping a disk to straining muscles, or even dropping dead! Are there any 'commandments' that I should be following?

Follow these guidelines.

- Never exercise until it hurts. If you begin to feel uncomfortable, stop immediately and rest.

- Don't be embarrassed to rest – it is your health that matters, not your image.

- Avoid exercise within 2 hours of a main meal. The output from your heart rises by 20% to cope with digestion, so exercising too soon could make you feel unwell.

- Don't exercise if you feel under the weather with a cold or flu, or when you feel 'too tired'.

Warning signs that you are doing too much include:

- pain in your chest;

- breathlessness;

- palpitations (see Chapter 6);

- faint feelings; or

- just not feeling 'right'.

Stop immediately, and next time reduce the amount of exercise you do, stepping up again a week later. If warning signs continue when you are exercising less, go and see your doctor.

I am recuperating from a severe heart attack. How can I tell when I am overdoing things?

It is best to join a local cardiac rehabilitation programme, and most hospitals have these now. If you have not been told about such a programme, ask your doctor if there is one near you – it is most likely to have been overlooked.

Ask your doctor or nurse to show you how to take your pulse (see Figure 10.2 on p. 291). It should be less than 100 beats per minute (bpm) before you start exercising, and not go faster than 200 bpm minus your age: so if you are aged 60, your heart rate should not exceed 140 bpm. If your heart rate (measured at your pulse) is consistently greater than 100 bpm before you start exercising, it is best to get the doctor to check you over to make sure that all is well. At first your heart rate will rise quickly on exercise, but it will rise more slowly as you get fitter. If the rate goes above your maximum target, slow down as this is a sign you are overdoing things : it is very easy to be too keen!

Is it really necessary to know my heart rate?

No, it's not essential but some people like it as a guide. It is quite in order to judge based on how you feel and whether you are breathing comfortably. The best exercise is a progressive programme with a gradual increase in exercise supervised or guided by a rehabilitation nurse or physiotherapist.

I can honestly say that I have never taken any exercise, but my doctor tells me that I need to do so if I do not want more heart problems. For how long should I exercise?

Only for about 15 minutes at first. Don't overdo things: gradually increase the time and build more exercise into your day.

- Can you climb two flights of stairs instead of using a lift?

- Do you really need the car or the bus for the half mile or kilometre to the shops?

- Can you park half a mile from the station or get off the bus a stop early, and then walk the rest of the way?

Ideally exercise should be built up to 30–40 minutes a day, five or more times a week.

How will exercise help me?

Exercise helps you in many ways.

- It improves your breathing and thus the supply of oxygen.

- It strengthens your heart's pumping action.

- As your fitness improves, your general well-being improves, along with greater self-confidence.

- Any bottled up stress tends to be released, relaxation and sleep will be improved, and overall lethargy and fatigue decreased.

- Exercise also helps you lose weight and improves your cholesterol levels.

Exercise is cheap – all that is needed is the will to do it and a good pair of shoes.

Diet

Should I be doing anything about what I eat?

There are two main things about your eating that can be improved: reducing your weight and lowering your fat intake (cholesterol). Both are important and are usually related, although some thin people can have high cholesterol levels, and some fat people can have normal cholesterol levels. See the section *Risks of high cholesterol levels* in Chapter 2, for more information about cholesterol and lipids, and what is involved.

I am absolutely miserable when I go on a slimming diet – it never works anyway. What is so wrong with being fat?

Being overweight throws a strain on your heart and causes your blood pressure to rise. Fat people are less mobile and have more pain in their bones and joints.

Losing weight sensibly (and not 'going on a diet') will benefit your heart and help keep your blood pressure normal. If you are overweight, losing weight may also help reduce the fats in your body. There are guidelines for your ideal weight (see Appendix 4). Losing weight is about changing your lifestyle and the amount of food you eat. It is not about becoming obsessed with food or going on crash diets. See Chapter 9 for more information about losing weight.

Would it help if I saw a dietitian?

Yes. Dietitians are extremely good at explaining which foods are best to eat, and they know how to advise different ethnic groups with specific dietary requirements. Ask for an appointment at the hospital or at your doctor's surgery.

My cholesterol was checked 2 weeks after my heart attack. It had gone right down, but my hospital doctor did not seem as pleased as I was. Why not?

After a heart attack, the cholesterol level will fall and return to your normal level after about 6–8 weeks. If it is tested on the day that you are admitted for the heart attack, this will be accurate too. Cholesterol measurements taken after the first 24 hours and up to 2 months after a heart attack are unreliable, tend to be low and therefore falsely reassuring. Whatever your cholesterol was, you will be placed on a statin (forever!) as the benefits are overwhelming. Your response will be checked to make sure that the dose is correct and that the targets have been reached (see the section *Risks of high cholesterol levels* in Chapter 2).

I have read a lot about what I should do, now that I am home after my heart attack, but there seems to be too much to do at once.

It may seem that way at first, but it is important that you change your lifestyle. Don't get obsessed by the need to change, tackle each point of the diet as suggested in Chapter 9, in a gradual way. Get the whole family into healthy eating – pick up any hints or tips from family and friends, or leaflets from your pharmacist.

Begin with the simple tasks of reducing sugar, switching puddings to fruit, snacking sensibly on fruit and not biscuits, and then gradually switching from saturated to unsaturated fats. See the section *Risks of high cholesterol levels* in Chapter 2 and then read Chapter 9.

5 | Heart failure

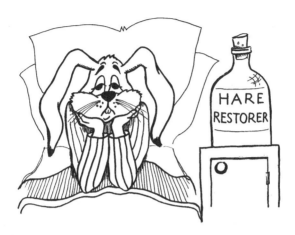

Heart failure occurs when the body's demands for energy are not supplied properly because of a weakness in the heart itself. Heart failure from damage to the heart muscle is common and, at present, 0.3% of the UK population is affected each year. However, it becomes more of a problem with increasing age, as it affects 8% of those over 65 years of age. Put another way, many thousands of people develop heart failure each year, and this represents 5% of acute emergency admissions to hospital. Because heart failure is common in elderly people, one of the reasons why we are seeing more cases of heart failure is the fact that people are living longer. In total up to 2% of the population actually suffers – roughly 1 million people in the UK. Each year 120 000 people are admitted to hospital with heart failure and stay on average 11 days. Heart failure costs the NHS over £300 million per year. Heart failure, if not treated, can significantly shorten life and reduce its quality but we now have means of helping people to live longer and feel better.

CAUSES

Are the causes of heart failure known?

Heart failure usually occurs because of a weakness of the heart muscle. The heart then doesn't pump as strongly as it should. The most common cause of damage to the muscle is a heart attack but it can also be due to:

- narrowing (hardening) of the coronary arteries;

- high blood pressure;

- narrow or leaking valves;

- a disease of the muscle itself (cardiomyopathy), where the muscle is affected directly, usually by a virus, and not as a consequence of other problems such as high blood pressure;

- excess alcohol consumption over many years.

My daughter has been diagnosed as having cardiomyopathy – what is this condition?

Cardiomyopathy (pronounced 'car-dee-oh-my-opathee') is a disease of the heart muscle. The muscles may be too thick – this is known as hypertrophic cardiomyopathy (*hypertrophy* means thickening) – or too thin and too weak so that the heart enlarges and looks flabby (doctors often call this a 'saggy bag' heart). Both conditions can cause heart failure. The commonest is the weak heart and the medical term for this is *congestive cardiomyopathy*. Hypertrophic cardiomyopathy is usually inherited and can be the cause of sudden death in apparently fit young people. Although coronary disease can weaken the heart muscle, your daughter's diagnosis of cardiomyopathy is probably related to disease of the heart muscle even though she has normal coronary arteries.

I have read of footballers and other sports people dropping dead from HOCM – what is this?

Hypertrophic cardiomyopathy (see above question) can cause so much thickening of the heart muscle that it obstructs the flow of blood leaving the heart. It then becomes Hypertrophic Obstructive Cardiomyopathy or HOCM. This obstruction is increased when physical exercise or strong emotion increases the heart rate. It can then block the flow of blood or cause the heart's electric system to become so irregular from lack of oxygen that the person collapses (we call this *syncope* – sudden loss of consciousness). Sadly, this collapse can be out of the blue and fatal. If the problem can be detected earlier, treatments are available with medication to help prevent a collapse. People with HOCM should be managed in specialised units to allow for optimal care, as it is not a straightforward condition.

How often do sports players collapse and die?

Hypertrophic cardiomyopathy affects one in 500 people and along with other very rare conditions, it is estimated that 0.2% of the athletic population may have a problem with the heart that could affect them at some time. Deaths during sports have been estimated at between one in 100 000 and one in 300 000 in young athletes. However, in older people, because of the increased chance of having coronary disease, the death rate varies from one in 15 000 for joggers to one in 50 000 for marathon runners. Dramatic and newsworthy death during sports is rare. Currently, the Football Association is using some of its income from TV coverage to screen all young would-be football stars by ECG and echocardiography – a commendable approach to safety in the sport.

My husband has heart failure but the doctor says his heart is OK, he's just anaemic. How can this be?

The heart can fail because of other problems. If there isn't enough blood (through anaemia or blood loss, e.g. after an accident), the heart will overwork until it fails, because there is so little blood to pump around. It may also fail if the thyroid gland is overactive (*thyrotoxicosis*) because an overactive thyroid gland drives the heart very fast and can cause it to go into atrial fibrillation (see Chapter 6). Usually the heart recovers when the conditions are treated.

If the heart valves are to blame for weakened muscle, can they be replaced?

Yes. An operation to replace defective heart valves is a successful way of relieving heart failure, providing the heart muscles (the 'pump') are not too severely damaged (see Chapter 7).

I have been told that I have heart failure. Is heart failure dangerous?

It can be if not treated properly. People with mild heart failure usually lead a normal life, but those with more severe heart failure will be restricted in what they can do: the weaker the heart, the greater the problem. The good news is that modern drugs, especially the ACE inhibitors (see the section *Treatment* below), can add many high quality years to the life of anyone with heart failure. If you have heart failure, ask your doctor about ACE inhibitors if you are not taking them – they are very important drugs, and can help you a lot.

SYMPTOMS

What are the symptoms of heart failure?

When your heart does not pump enough blood around the body, fluid builds up because there is not enough energy to push the fluid through the kidneys into your bladder. The medical word for a build-up of fluid is *oedema* (pronounced 'ee-dee-ma'). If the fluid builds up in your lungs, you become breathless, with a wheeze or a cough, and you may produce frothy sputum. If the fluid builds up around your ankles, they will swell up and you will be able to see indentations from your shoes or socks or from pressing your skin with a finger (be careful, it can be painful).

My partner has been diagnosed with heart failure but no one would guess on meeting her. However, she does get breathless at night. Why is this?

Fluid builds up in her lungs when she lies down and, if she is asleep, her defences are down. She may wake up with a suffocating feeling. This is helped by standing or sitting up, as this will take the pressure off her lungs. Some people open the window, feeling the need to gulp in fresh air, others walk around or go downstairs to make a cup of tea. If you can reassure her that all is well, this will help her to keep calm. She should tell her doctor that this is happening as medication can help to relieve it.

I have heart failure. Am I right to be worried that I will not be able to lead an active life?

Patients with minimal heart failure usually have no limitations to ordinary physical activity. Mild heart failure leads to breathlessness on walking a mile on the flat, one or two flights of stairs or a long incline. Moderate heart failure tends to cause symptoms more readily – walking half a mile on the flat or one flight of stairs leads to needing a rest. Severe heart failure causes breathlessness on minimal effort and even at rest. Everyone is different, so personal issues are usually best discussed with your doctor.

The good news is that we have treatments that can relieve or at least improve any symptoms so that a better exercise ability and quality of life can be enjoyed. People with more severe symptoms have to learn to adapt their lifestyle once all treatments have been tried and they still remain limited. If you are overweight, reducing your weight can help by taking some of the workload off the weakened heart pump.

You will probably be able to go on holiday and travel as usual, but make your plans more carefully to avoid rushing to catch aeroplanes or trains. Discuss with your doctor if you are planning long journeys while you are on water tablets (see the section *Treatment* below) as these may need adjusting: dehydration can be a problem on long flights.

Sexual activity doesn't usually present a problem and is not harmful. As in all forms of exercise, breathlessness might limit what you can manage, so take advice if this occurs (see Chapter 8). Some tablets can make you lose your sexual drive and, if this has happened, you should mention this to your doctor rather than accept it. Your doctor may be able to change your medication. Remember, don't suddenly stop taking your medication as this could be dangerous.
People often keep to themselves their worries and anxieties. Don't do this – most of your problems can be alleviated: don't be afraid to let the doctor know what's on your mind.

> *I had a heart attack recently. My cardiologist tells me that my heart has weakened and that I have now got heart failure. Will the symptoms be noticeable?*

Your weight may go up from the retention of fluid (1 kg = 1 litre or 1 lb = 1 pint). Your doctor will monitor treatment by measuring your weight loss after you have been prescribed diuretics (these are pills to make you pass more water). There are other symptoms that you might notice:

- feeling tired and washed out;

- swollen ankles ('I can't get my usual shoes on');

- swollen tummy (so your clothing is tight); and

- on occasions, you may get a bit confused.

My doctor says I have a hibernating myocardium. What does he mean?

Your heart muscle looks weak and damaged but is capable of getting a lot of its power back; the damage is not irreversible. The heart is literally hibernating. If your heart only appears to be damaged, it may be possible to strengthen it by angioplasty or surgery. If that is possible, your quality of life and length of life will be greatly improved.

The doctor will check your heart to see what its strength is, either with an echocardiogram, perhaps a nuclear (thallium) scan, or a technique known as positron emission tomography (PET for short). See the section *Tests* below.

Should I discuss the diagnosis of heart failure with my family?

It is always important with any illness to discuss its effects with close family and friends and, if appropriate, workmates. Having heart failure may limit you because of breathlessness, fatigue and weakness. Your family and friends will be worried about you – by bringing them into the picture they will be able to help and support you.

TESTS

It is important to know the cause of heart failure because, if it is mechanical (such as a leaking valve), you will need a mechanical solution (a new valve). If it is heart muscle failure, you will need tablets. A high blood pressure will need urgent treatment. Investigations sort this out. Usually you will have an ECG (see Chapter 2), a chest X-ray, blood tests and an echocardiogram. These are all discussed below.

The doctor at the hospital told me that I have heart failure. For some reason, he told me to report back for a chest X-ray. Why do I need a chest X-ray for heart failure?

An X-ray picture of your chest will tell him about the size of your heart and its shape; this will help the doctor work out the cause of your heart failure. He will also get a picture of your lungs and can tell whether there is any infection or fluid there.

You will be asked to stand in front of an X-ray plate, and then told to breathe in and hold your breath for a few seconds. As you hold your breath, the picture is taken. Holding your breath will prevent a blurred image occurring. The X-ray dose is very small and not in any way dangerous.

Why do I need blood tests for heart failure?

Your doctor will need to make sure that you are not anaemic, as this can make heart failure worse (see earlier question). Your kidney function will also be checked and any evidence of a congested liver looked for. Blood may also be taken to make sure that your thyroid gland is not under- or overactive. Any evidence of liver damage from alcohol will be monitored. Liver congestion is not unusual in heart failure and improves rapidly with treatment. A test for Brain Naturetic Peptide (BNP) is frequently performed and elevated levels identify heart failure.

My sister is very concerned that she has been given an appointment to have an echocardiogram. What is this?

This is a painless, simple test which tells us about the size of her heart, how well it is working, how strong the muscle is and how the valves are working. It is often used to assess the significance of a heart murmur and the size of a heart attack, to see if any clots are forming and to calculate the efficiency of the heart's muscle pump.

How is an echocardiogram performed?

The room, in a hospital or at your family doctor's, is usually darkened to allow the doctor or technician (cardiac physiologist) to see the screen. You may be asked to lie on your back or side (see Figure 5.1). A special type of jelly is put on your chest and a probe applied to the jelly. The probe is moved over your chest. Ultrasound waves (it is not an X-ray being taken) are bounced off your heart and a picture of the heart's movements and structure made.

You are usually able to see what is happening and the pictures are stored on video or disc which the doctor may show you. It usually takes 20 minutes and is painless, with no side effects.

Doppler ultrasound is also used and this measures the blood flow. It makes a noise like a washing machine.

My doctor wants a special echocardiogram to see if I might benefit from a pacemaker. What is this about?

A new treatment for heart failure is a special pacemaker which is used when the two heart pumps are out of synchrony, that is, not beating at the same time. A special echo measures the dysynchrony index. If this is abnormal, it suggests that the heart can be brought back in line with a cardiac re-synchrony pacemaker. The efficiency of the heart will be improved and you will feel better. Sometimes this special pacemaker will be combined with a defibrillator which may prevent you dying suddenly.

I have heard that some echocardiograms are done by the patient swallowing a tube. Is this true and, if so, what is happening here?

Yes, it is true. The reason is that your gullet is situated behind the heart, and a scan from the gullet (or *oesophagus*, pronounced 'ee-sof-a-gus') gives better pictures than one on the chest, when the probe has to steer round the lungs. This is known as *transoesophageal* (via your food pipe) *echocardiography* (TOE or TEE in America). It is done when we need specialised additional information, particularly on valve or clot problems. The tube is not large and is usually passed after you have been given relaxing medication and a local spray anaesthetic

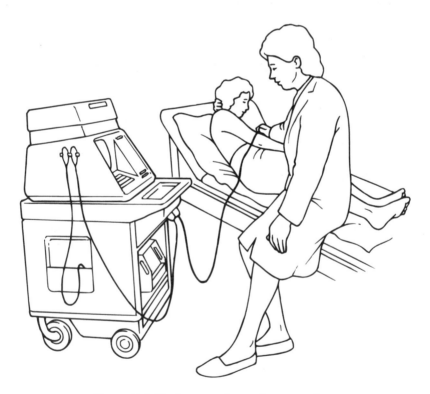

Figure 5.1 Having an echocardiogram taken.

to the mouth. Some people do find it unpleasant but it is a very important test to help guide your treatment.

I have an appointment at the hospital for a nuclear scan. This sounds rather dangerous to me. Is it harmful and how is a nuclear scan done?

The radioactive levels are low and not at all dangerous – you won't glow in the dark! A scanning machine takes pictures of your heart following an injection of a radioactive material (usually thallium or sestamibi) into a vein. If your heart is healthy, the thallium is absorbed and an even picture will be shown. If there is damage to your heart, the thallium will not be taken up well by the bits of your heart that are not working efficiently. If there is scar tissue from a heart attack, there will be a gap or a hole in the picture as no thallium will be taken up. If your heart is made to work hard by an exercise test or by the injection of a stimulant to speed it up, the thallium will not travel well to any areas where there is a poor blood supply (such as in that caused by coronary narrowing). When your heart rests between beats and the demand for blood falls, thallium can reach this area. In this way, the scanner can give a very accurate and useful picture to your doctor. First it shows a deficit, but then shows whether this deficit can be rectified. If the scanner shows a hole in the picture which does not improve, then it is likely that the muscle is dead and cannot be improved.

The hospital has written to me and told me that I need a test called a SPECT. What is this?

This is *single photon emission computed tomography*. It is a 3-D scanning system. You will lie on a table and the scanner rotates to take pictures from different angles, again helping to identify damaged muscle or muscle suffering from a lack of blood supply. It is a sophisticated test but simple to do – like a standard sestamibi scan but with bells on!

I have had test after test until I feel that I could not be tested further. I now have been summoned for a nuclear scan. When is nuclear scanning specifically helpful?

Nuclear scanning can be very useful for people with angina, after a heart attack and when there is heart failure. It is a means of trying to assess the importance of each narrowing present, and whether any good can be done by treatment. It is more expensive than an exercise test but useful when exercise tests cannot be done (for instance if you have arthritis), or when specific information on your heart muscle is needed that a treadmill exercise test cannot provide.

My wife was told that she is going to have a PET scan. How is PET different from SPECT?

PET is *positron emission tomography* and this is a very specialised technique involving nuclear scanning, and it accurately tells us about blood flow and whether the heart muscle is hibernating or not. It is a very expensive test, so is used only when really necessary. It can, however, identify where help might be possible when other tests have not been able to show what can done; so, used carefully, it represents value for money.

TREATMENT

I have been told that I have heart failure but was also informed that I will not need treatment for some time; why not? And, if I have to have treatment in the future, what might it consist of?

First of all, the tests will decide on the cause of your heart failure. A high blood pressure, coronary artery disease, severe lung damage, excess alcohol and problems with the valves are all possible causes. A leaking valve may be repaired or replaced; a narrow valve can be replaced or stretched by a large balloon (see Chapter 7), and a big scar from a heart attack, which causes the muscle to stretch (*aneurysm*, pronounced 'ann-ure-ism'), can be cut out. Most of the time the problem is likely to involve the muscle pump and your treatment then is with tablets (see Box).

DRUGS FOR HEART FAILURE

Diuretics (water pills)
    amiloride
    bendroflumethiazide
    bumetanide
    furosemide
    spironolactone

Angiotensin converting enzyme inhibitors
    captopril
    cilazapril
    enalapril
    fosinopril
    lisinopril
    perindopril
    quinapril
    ramipril
    trandolapril

Digoxin

Nitrates
    isosorbide dinitrate
    isosorbide mononitrate

Beta-blockers
    bisoprolol
    carvedilol
    metoprolol

Angiotensin II antagonists
    candesartan
    irbesartan
    losartan
    valsartan

Sinus node slowers
    ivabradine

I have had an unpleasant jolt, having a heart attack. I suppose that I ignored the advice and warnings. Now I am determined not to lose control again. My doctor says it's heart failure. What can I do to help myself with my heart problem?

The main thing is to guard against increasing the fluid build-up in your body (in your lungs or legs particularly). Therefore:

- try to lose weight;

- keep as active as you can;

- avoid salty foods or adding salt at the table;

- weigh yourself every day to check to see if you have put on weight which might be due to increased fluid;

- take your medicine as directed;

- keep in touch with your support nurse for advice.

If you find it harder to breathe, your ankles puff up, or you feel generally washed out, go and see your doctor. Don't let the fluid build up too much as it alters the absorption of some medications making treatment more difficult.

Medication

I have been prescribed diuretics. What are these?

Diuretics are commonly known as water tablets. They act to stimulate the kidney to get rid of the excess fluid which causes breathlessness and swollen ankles. Some tablets, such as furosemide and bumetanide, act quickly: you will notice that you need to go to the toilet a lot over the first four hours or so after you have taken the tablet. This occurs every time you take the tablets but is usually over with by six hours. You need to plan when to take the tablets, so that you are not caught short. Some, the thiazides, are milder and gentler than others and these help to spread the passing of water over a 10–12 hour period.

Most diuretics flush potassium out of the body and this may need to be replaced by tablets. Blood tests will help the doctor keep an eye on the chemicals in your blood. Doctors measure the 'urea and electrolytes' levels in a blood sample; these levels monitor your kidney function, potassium and sodium (you can remember them as 'electric lights'). In addition, as estimated glomerular filtration rate (eGFR) is now routinely calculated to monitor kidney function more precisely.

How will I know if the diuretics are working?

You will be able to breathe better and your ankles will be less swollen. Your weight will go down as the fluid is urinated out. If your weight goes up, you will need more water pills but, if it drops too low, you may need them reducing, as you may have got rid of too much fluid. We try to use the lowest doses possible.

Sometimes the tablets don't work and the drugs have to be temporarily given by an injection in a vein. This usually needs specialised treatment in a hospital. Once the fluid levels have been controlled, the tablets will be started again and this usually keeps the fluid at bay.

My doctor tells me that I need digoxin to help my heart. Why?

Digoxin is a tablet which in some people helps regulate an irregular heartbeat (*atrial fibrillation*: see Chapter 6) and makes the heart more efficient. It is also used to strengthen the heart muscle, giving it more pumping power. If the drug builds up too much in your blood, it can cause loss of appetite and nausea. Your doctor may check the level of digoxin in the blood with a blood test and adjust the dose to get the best effect without side effects.

My doctor has taken me off water tablets and put me on ACE inhibitors, which don't agree with me at all – they just make me cough all the time. Why?

ACE inhibitors stands for angiotensin-converting enzyme inhibitors. These are very important medicines that, in some people, increase their ability to exercise, as well as reducing breathlessness and fatigue. People will feel better on this medication and their life can be prolonged. Side effects are not common but occasionally people get a dry hacking cough. This is more common in women and Chinese people. If your cough is a problem (and is not due to fluid), ACE inhibitors can be switched to AII antagonists (see under

Treatment in the section *Risks of high blood pressure* in Chapter 2) which have similar effects without producing the cough. Research studies show they are very effective drugs and may improve treatment by being prescribed in addition to ACE inhibitors as well as an alternative if ACE inhibitors cannot be tolerated. Studies with candesartan and valsartan have given impressive results, which are probably applicable to the other AII drugs.

Generally, doctors try to get everyone with heart failure to take ACE inhibitors if at all possible. ACE inhibitors are prescribed with diuretics and have the advantage of retaining the potassium that the diuretics wash out. They are quite often prescribed with diuretics and digoxin. Commonly used ACE inhibitors are captopril, enalapril, lisinopril, ramipril and perindopril.

It is likely that more people will be on ACE inhibitors or AII drugs either alone, or in combination, as the research suggests patients with mild failure do not develop a more severe condition and overall well-being is improved.

My wife has heart failure and gets very breathless. She was prescribed nitrates at her last visit to the doctor. What are these for?

Nitrate tablets (isosorbide mononitrate or dinitrate) are sometimes used to help breathlessness, particularly if heart failure and angina occur together. Although the treatment is effective, headaches can be a limiting side effect (see the section *Treatment* in Chapter 3).

I have been prescribed warfarin. I thought this was rat poison! Why am I taking it?

Warfarin is a blood-thinning medicine and is used to prevent clot formation if your heartbeat is irregular (*atrial fibrillation*: see Chapter 6) or if the echocardiogram shows something that might mean you may develop clots. It may kill rats but for you it helps prevent a stroke. Warfarin reacts with many medicines and alcohol, so make sure you get a list of these drugs from your doctor. Regular sensible alcohol intake should not be harmful as the reaction between warfarin and alcohol will be constant, but drinking in bouts, or heavily, is dangerous as it may not only disturb the warfarin control but further damage the heart. Heart failure caused by alcohol means that you will have to stop drinking alcohol completely – the heart may improve as a result.

The effects of warfarin need to be monitored with regular blood tests. The INR (International Normalised Ratio) is a test for measuring the thinness of blood – normal is 1. On warfarin, the INR should be between 2.0 and 3.0. In some people the INR varies a lot for no obvious reason and blood tests have to be frequent for accurate monitoring. When the blood is stable, the test may be monthly or less frequent.

Machines are available to allow you to test and monitor yourself at home.

Should I be taking aspirin? I have heard a lot about it in the media recently.

Aspirin may be used instead of warfarin, particularly in milder cases of heart failure or when the heart rhythm is regular (normal sinus rhythm, not atrial fibrillation). The dose is 75 mg daily. Aspirin can upset the stomach so you may prefer to take the soluble form in a glass of water or with food. Coated aspirin (such as Nu-seals) is available and may help protect the stomach if regular soluble aspirin upsets you. Clopidogrel 75 mg daily is an alternative.

Can I take other medicines while I am on any of these heart failure tablets?

Other medicines may be used for specific problems. Ask your doctor or chemist if there is any chance of a reaction. Do not take arthritis pills without first discussing them with your doctor, as they can interact with heart failure medication. Some antacids contain salt so ask the chemist about the choices available.

Should I be taking beta-blockers?

In the past, the response would have been a firm no. Now research has shown that, once the failure has been controlled, beta-blockers may improve both symptoms and length of survival. Dosage is very low to start with, and under hospital supervision. When starting beta-blockers, you may not feel as good at first but, after a week or two, you should gradually feel better.

I have heart failure – can you tell me which drugs I should be taking and why?

Yes. The list below should help (see also the box **Drugs for Heart Failure** on p. 181). Your doctor may prescribe one of these or a combination.

- **Diuretics (water pills)** These reduce fluid and relieve breathlessness and ankle swelling.

- **ACE inhibitors** Used to improve the heart's pumping efficacy and improve life expectancy.

- **Warfarin** Used in atrial fibrillation and some other irregular heartbeats to reduce clots.

- **Digoxin** Used to help control atrial fibrillation and, in some severe cases in normal sinus rhythm, to improve symptoms.

- **Beta-blockers** Used to improve symptoms and length of survival.

- **AII antagonists** Used in cases where ACE inhibitors cause a cough, and in combination.

- **Statins** Used to reduce cholesterol when coronary disease is also present.

I recently read about spironolactone. Will this be given to me?

Spironolactone is an old diuretic (water pill). In a study of more severe cases, when it was added to diuretics, such as furosemide and ACE inhibitors, further improvement was noted. A problem arose in that the ACE inhibitors were used in lower doses than usually recommended, so we are unclear as to the exact benefit. If ACE inhibitors cannot be used or increased in dose because of side effects, spironolactone should certainly be considered.

My doctor placed me on eplerenone because I developed heart failure after a heart attack. How does it work?

It works like spironolactone, antagonising a hormone call aldosterone which becomes elevated in heart failure causing fluid retention. It helps prevent potassium loss, so like spironolactone needs to be carefully monitored with blood tests if used with ACE inhibitors or AII antagonists. It has been shown to improve length of survival when started 3–14 days after a heart attack when there is evidence of heart failure. Spironolactone can cause swollen breasts in men which may be tender and eplerenone avoids this.

Can I help monitor my heart failure at home?

The easiest way is to weigh yourself at the same time of day with no clothes on. The best time is first thing before breakfast. If you gain 1 kg, that is, 1 litre of fluid (2 pints), this points to the need to increase your diuretics. If you gain weight 2 days on the run, ask your doctor for advice. If you have been given a weight plan already, follow the instructions regarding extra diuretics (water pills). Your weight should return to the baseline – if it does not, visit your doctor.

Surgery

I have been diagnosed as having heart failure. Will I be able to have a heart transplant?

If your heart muscle is very weak and your activity remains very limited in spite of optimal medical treatment, transplantation is the best option available to give you a better quality and length of life. You must be aged less than 60 years and you will need to be mentally strong and have support and help available. Some people will not be suitable because of other serious illnesses or problems.

What does a heart transplant involve?

If you have been placed on a waiting list, you must be available within 2–3 hours of being called because the donor heart can only be transplanted within 6 hours of the death of the donor. You will usually be given a beeper or mobile phone. The donor heart should be of the same blood group and match yours, as well as matching your immune system. The race and sex of the donor and recipient do not matter but the size of the heart should be similar to yours, although it does not need to be exactly the same.

The operation is performed on the bypass machine. The diseased heart is removed by separating it from all the vessels connected to it but the back walls of the right and left atria are left in place. The new heart is then stitched onto the vessels and the atria, and the bypass is discontinued to allow the new heart to take over (see Figure 5.2).

After the transplant, which is a straightforward procedure, you will stay in hospital for 2–3 weeks whilst drugs are used to suppress rejection of the new heart. Biopsies via a small catheter are taken from the heart to look for signs of rejection. This is a simple, painless procedure performed under a local anaesthetic and uses a vein in the neck. You will remain on drugs always to keep rejection at bay, and you need to watch your lifestyle carefully: hardening of the arteries in the new heart is a particular problem and is checked for at regular

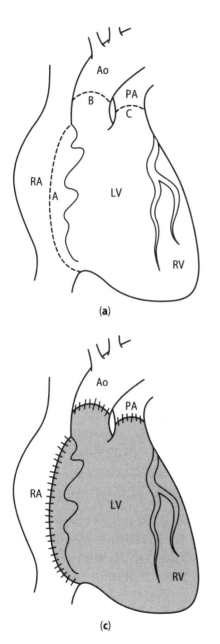
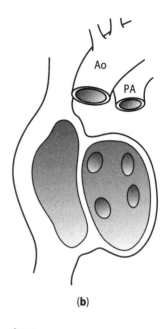

Ao = Aorta
PA = Pulmonary artery
RA = Right atrium
LV = Left ventricle
RV = Right ventricle

Figure 5.2 Heart transplant operation. (**a**) Heart being removed, with cuts at A, B and C; (**b**) no heart in place; (**c**) new heart stitched on.

intervals by your transplant doctor. A transplant that is successful will transform your life. After 1 year, 8 out of 10 patients will still be alive, and 6 out of 10 will live beyond 5 years.

I've heard about an operation to reduce the size of the heart by cutting out a piece of heart muscle. It is claimed to help heart failure. Should I consider this before a transplant?

This is a debated operation. In many of the cases, a new mitral valve is also put in, so that it is difficult to sort out which part of the operation has been successful. It must remain a part of a careful evaluation programme before it is widely used. We need to know the risk of death at the time of the operation and if the operation works – for how long and what evidence there is for improved quality of life. It is still in its early phase of evaluation when caution should replace over-enthusiasm.

My doctor has mentioned cardiomyoplasty but was not very enthusiastic about it. What is this operation?

This was an idea for surgery for the failing heart. A large muscle taken from a patient's back was loosened and then wrapped around the heart. A pacemaker was used to stimulate the muscle to squeeze the heart and give it more power. Initial enthusiasm has been replaced with disappointment as any benefit did not last long.

Is an artificial heart another option for me?

It may be a short-term help, if the heart is severely inflamed by a virus, when it might buy time for recovery. It might also buy time for a transplant donor to be found. At present, it does not offer a long-term solution, but it acts as a bridge to definitive therapy.

Can pacemakers be used to treat heart failure?

Pacemakers are usually used if there is an electrical fault with the heart (see the section *How your heart works* in Chapter 1). However, a special pacing technique has been developed for heart failure, which can be used even if the electrical connections are intact. It is used in more severe cases but is not suitable for everyone. Results have been very encouraging and it is certainly a treatment to consider. It is called resynchronisation therapy.

My cardiologist has advised a defibrillator as well as a pacemaker. Why both?

It is one combined unit. The pacemaker improves the heart's efficiency and the defibrillator stops dangerous, life-threatening changes in heart rhythm by giving the heart a shock. It is recommended when heart failure is more severe or when dangerous rhythms have already occurred. It is inserted by cardiologists who specialise in electrical events affecting the heart, and regular follow-up checks are needed.

6 | Palpitations

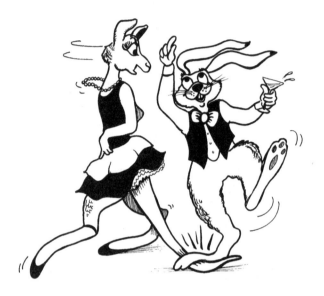

The medical word for palpitations is *arrhythmia* (pronounced 'ay-rith-me-ar') meaning a change in the beating rhythm of the heart.

All of us feel the heart pounding away when we have to run for a bus, have seen an exciting film or had a fright: this is the normal response to exertion or excitement which causes the adrenaline in the blood to increase and stimulate the heart to beat faster. Being aware of the heartbeat, when there is no obvious explanation, can be alarming and lead to anxiety and panic, all of which makes the situation worse.

What doctors mean by palpitations is an undue awareness of the heartbeat. People see it in less matter-of-fact terms: 'missed beats', 'big beats', 'pounding', 'fluttering', 'as if my heart was going to jump out of my chest' are some of my patients' descriptions. Underlying these sensations the questions really bothering people are:

- Am I going to die?

- Will I have a heart attack?

- Will my heart stop beating?

- Will it damage me?

First, it is very rare for any form of palpitations to be dangerous or life-threatening. It is true that they are frightening and the fear can make them worse, but, for most people, all they have to fear is the fear, because palpitations do not usually mean disease.

For the vast majority of people, palpitations are just one of the ways that stresses and strains on the body show themselves, so they tend to be more common in people experiencing stress at home or work, in those with family anxieties and in those who are run down or overworked.

TYPES OF PALPITATIONS

I often feel that my heart has missed a beat. Is this serious?

Missed beats are a common sort of palpitation and are invariably harmless. They can be brought on by too much caffeine, for example in tea, coffee, Coca-Cola or chocolate. Of these, coffee is by far the most important source of caffeine. Sometimes alcohol is the cause. If there is another disease present, missed beats may well be important, for example after a heart attack (see your doctor if you get these), but in 9 out of 10 people the heart is sound.

I drink rather a lot of coffee. I have heard that caffeine is bad for the heart and I must admit that sometimes I feel that my heart has missed a beat. Am I about to have a heart attack?

The control of the heart is like an electric circuit with a master switch. Occasionally, short circuits cause extra beats but the master switch is always in charge, even though it lets one or two extra beats escape. You may feel this more when your heart is slow, or when you are resting or just before going to sleep. It can also occur when the heart has been stimulated by caffeine, alcohol, stress, or as a side effect of medication, such as inhalers for asthma. The extra beat arrives early and there is then a pause (the missed beat) whilst the next normal beat comes along. The extra beat may not be felt ('as if the heart skips a beat') but, after the pause, the pump of the heart will be fuller than usual, so the next normal beat will feel like a big beat – a 'kick' or a 'thump'. A beat hasn't really been missed, it just feels like it, and the big beat is the heart making up for the one that came a bit early. This is not dangerous – the heart is compensating for the early beat.

When I was at work the other day, I suddenly felt my heart was working overtime – I hadn't even been rushing up the stairs! What was happening?

Rapid palpitations may be normal, such as when you are running or excited, but sometimes they occur abruptly ('out of the blue') and can cause mainly fear, but also a sweaty feeling, light-headedness, breathlessness or, rarely, pain. Just as the cause of extra beats can be thought of as short circuits, so these palpitations are best thought of as caused by a sensitive area in the wiring of your heart. Again, it may be responding to stress, cigarettes, caffeine or alcohol. Remember that the wiring is only part of the building of the heart, a problem here or there is not going to affect the structure. However, palpitations which lead to chest pain, light-headedness or blackouts need a thorough medical check, so go to your doctor if you get these symptoms. Some people – a small number – have persistent troublesome rapid palpitations which carry on even when you have stopped drinking caffeine or alcohol or when you are no longer stressed. The cause can invariably be identified and treated and is rarely more than an awkward nuisance. Although there may be no major problem with the heart, there is no point in feeling ill if treatment can help you.

I've been very worried when I had two attacks of rapid heartbeats recently. Are there any types of palpitations that are dangerous?

Some very rare palpitations are so fast that a blackout occurs. If they occur because your heart muscle is not working very well (*ventricular tachycardia* – tachycardia just means rapid heartbeat), you will need medication to make them stop as they can be fatal. A common medication used is amiodarone. Your doctor will explain what is happening and it will be very important to follow his advice. You will need close hospital supervision. A defibrillator may also be advised (see p. 191). I must emphasise that this is rare.

I am in my twenties and am getting rapid heartbeats every so often. I work in the type of job where results are all important. My husband has just lost his job as well, so sometimes I feel really stressed. Should I go to the doctor?

Rapid palpitations are a bit more of a problem because they are more scary. Again, younger people can be under stress, and the heart is behaving in an exaggerated variation of normal, as if you are running all the time, owing to higher adrenaline levels in the blood. A visit to your doctor and an ECG are necessary if symptoms are a problem (dizziness, breathlessness). The doctor will test you for various things such as anaemia, an overactive thyroid gland; he may also check to see whether you are pregnant, because pregnancy makes the heart beat faster in order to feed the baby. Very rarely, the ECG shows evidence of a specific 'extra wire' in the heart, which conducts beats much faster than the usual circuit; you will need to go to hospital in this case.

SELF-HELP

I occasionally get palpitations. Now that I am approaching 50 are they going to get worse?

The first thing to do is not to panic. Your doctor will have already told you about not smoking and not drinking excess caffeine or alcohol. As you get older it is a good idea also to try and keep your weight down. Make sure that you:

- take regularly any tablets you have been prescribed;
- attend your doctor for regular checks;
- report any change in how you feel.

I have just had three attacks of palpitations in a week, which made me very worried. By the time I got to see my doctor, they had gone away. What should I do if I get another attack?

When you experience palpitations, take deep breaths and try to relax. If you feel faint, sit down or lie down with your feet up. Try doing a deep cough. If the palpitations are missed beats or rapid beats, and you feel unwell or know that you have a heart condition, let your doctor know. If you are otherwise well and just afraid, ask yourself whether any of these factors might have caused it:

- stress;
- caffeine;
- workload;
- alcohol;
- smoking;
- family anxiety or grief;

- problems at work;

- no recent holiday;

- being generally run-down and anxious.

Try to help yourself by learning to relax more and avoid stimulants to the heart.

After you have tried the first-line principles of not panicking, taking deep breaths etc., try the following procedures, designed to stimulate a nerve called the vagus nerve which can switch rapid palpitations off. These include:

- drinking ice-cold liquid or eating ice-cream, or putting your hand in a bucket of cold water;

- coughing deeply;

- blowing your nose with it pinched, as if trying to make your ears pop, for 20 seconds;

- pressing the right artery in the neck (this is known as carotid sinus massage (CSM) and needs medical instruction);

Do not press your eyes as this can be dangerous.

If rapid palpitations are a more frequent problem or cause distressing symptoms, then medication will be needed to suppress them (see the section *Treatment* below). Many types are available and more than one may be necessary. Just because you may need more than one medication does not mean that palpitations are dangerous, just awkward. Treatment is a bit hit and miss, so be patient and ask your doctor about any side effects.

I have heart disease and am finding that I occasionally get attacks of palpitations. Is this serious?

Missed beats in people with heart disease are not usually much to worry about but a check-up is a good idea. Those people on water pills (diuretics – see the question on diuretics in the section *Risks of high blood pressure* in Chapter 2), or blood pressure pills (see Chapter 2) may have a low potassium level. Although this is not a common cause of missed beats, the problem can easily be treated, so it should be considered if palpitations arise for no obvious reason when these medications are being taken. You should ask your doctor if your palpitations seem to arise for no apparent reason. Fresh fruit contains lots of potassium as does fruit juice, so the treatment is pleasant; however, it is best to avoid grapefruit juice as this affects the action of some medications.

There was something in the media about a problem with grapefruit juice interacting in some way with medications. Should I avoid the fruit or juice completely?

It is the concentrated juice that is a problem. The juice leaves the body via the liver where it shares the same breakdown system as some medications. It competes with the medications and stops them from being broken down (*metabolised*) so they may stay around much longer than normal and become more powerful.

I am in my sixties and have developed rapid heartbeats in the last few weeks. I like to drink with friends most evenings. Do you think I am drinking too much?

Rapid palpitations in older people may be caused by atrial fibrillation (see below). This is an irregular heartbeat caused by wear and tear but it is also more common in people with high blood pressure and those who drink a lot of alcohol. Sometimes it can be due to the coronary arteries becoming narrowed or to a thyroid problem (*thyrotoxicosis*).

If the rapid palpitations are other than normal speeding up (*sinus tachycardia*), your doctor may decide to treat you and base the treatment on how you feel. For instance, if your heart is sound and only one attack a month happens, then the main thing for you to do will be to cut down on your drinking which acts as a stimulant. Your doctor may treat you for high blood pressure.

I have tried all sorts of self-help methods but I keep getting palpitation attacks; when should I see the doctor?

Palpitations are common, mostly harmless but invariably worrying. Don't be afraid, try to understand the reasons – have a good look at how you are living and seek medical advice if there is not an obvious cause or the attacks just won't go away. If palpitations lead to symptoms of chest pain, light-headedness or blackouts, always get your doctor to check you over.

TESTS

I have been to the doctor because I was so worried about these rapid heartbeats that occurred. He has given me a little machine to record any attacks that I get in future. Can you tell me more about this please?

Because palpitations don't usually occur when you visit the doctor, a 24-hour ECG (see Chapter 2) is often used. This is like a 'Walkman' but it records your heartbeats instead of playing music. The digital card is replayed through a computer and we see the results in a matter of minutes. It does not record any sound so you need not worry that Big Brother is listening in!

You can use this machine at home so that the doctors can watch what your heart is doing during normal daily life. You will be asked to keep a diary and the recording will be checked for times when you felt palpitations or became dizzy.

Four electrodes are attached to your chest and fastened with wires to the recorder which is worn on a belt round your waist (see Figure 6.1). The monitor is quiet and you should not be inconvenienced.

Whilst using the recorder, act normally and try to bring on the symptoms you have been having. You are not allowed to have a bath or shower without a special cover being used. You will be asked to return the recorder the next day so that we can analyse the recording to see if you need any special treatment. Sometimes we do several recordings over 2–5 days.

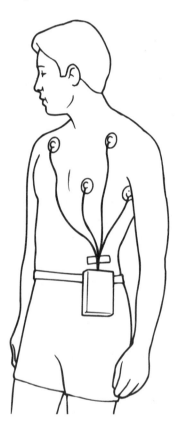

Figure 6.1 A mobile ECG recorder known as a Holter, about the size of a 'Walkman'.

I think the machine that I am to be given is called an event recorder. Is this different to the 'Walkman'-type recorder?

This is a small machine which you put on your chest to record a palpitation as it happens. It is about the size of a mobile phone and can be carried easily. The palpitation is then decoded over the telephone or in the technicians' department, and printed out on an ECG. It is useful when attacks are infrequent but noticeable, and they have to be long enough for you to take action to record them. You will be shown how to use it by the technician at the outpatient department when you collect it.

There are now several recorders which you can activate yourself – some are very small so they are easy to live with. They store information which can then be downloaded and analysed on a computer. They are particularly useful when attacks are infrequent, and where a 24-hour ECG may miss them. Sometimes a device called a Reveal is inserted under the skin, under local anaesthetic. This is about the size of a PP3 battery and can be used to record infrequent episodes, being kept in place for up to a year.

An appointment has been made for me to go to hospital for electrophysiological (EPS) tests. What are these?

These are tests which have to be done in hospital, not at home. Pacemaker catheters (usually four) are passed via a vein at the top of your leg to the heart and the source of palpitations pinpointed and analysed with complex computers. It usually takes up to an hour but can take several hours; it generally needs to be done with X-ray guidance in the catheter laboratory. The only pain you should feel is the local anaesthetic in the groin, but as the doctor moves the catheters you may become aware of your palpitations as the doctor identifies them and tries to get them to occur again. It is usually done as a day case, or one night in hospital may be advised.

TREATMENT

*I have a very stressful job and find that I get really nervous.
My heart seems to miss a beat when I am stressed or anxious.
Is there anything that can help me?*

Missed beats usually respond to self-help, perhaps with a doctor's
reassurance which might include taking an ECG at rest and
recording the heartbeat for 24 hours (24-hour ECG see the section
Tests above). A lot of people, who get palpitations like this, are young
and under stress, and are helped by beta-blockers which block the
stimulation of adrenaline and caffeine to the heart (see the question
on beta-blockers in the section *Risks of high blood pressure* in
Chapter 2). These can be used for a month while you try and change
your lifestyle where possible, and then as required, for instance before
a stressful meeting. Try not to drink too much coffee at meetings and
change to decaffeinated-type drinks.

*I am going for tests at the hospital next week for palpitations.
Will I be offered any medication to treat irregular heartbeats?*

It will depend on what type of palpitations that you are found to
have. There are a large number of medications used to slow down
fast heartbeats and to suppress extra beats.

- **Digoxin** is most often used to control atrial fibrillation (see
  below). Doses vary according to how old you are and how good
  your kidneys are. Your body gets rid of digoxin through your
  kidneys so, if the kidney function is not as good as it should be,
  digoxin will build up in the blood. Commonest side effects are
  loss of appetite, nausea and vomiting. Your doctor may check
  the level of digoxin in the blood 6 hours after you have taken it
  to make sure it is not too high or too low. If you get side effects,
  these will probably disappear if the dose is reduced. (See the
  section *Treatment* in Chapter 5.)

- **Beta-blockers** are also used for controlling palpitations. They also help angina, heart failure and high blood pressure; they are especially useful if you have more than one of these conditions. (See under *Treatment* in the **Risks of high blood pressure** section in Chapter 2.)

- The **calcium antagonists**, verapamil and diltiazem, are alternatives to beta-blockers for palpitations and, like beta-blockers, can be combined with digoxin.

Other more specific medications can be used to suppress extra beats and these include flecainide and amiodarone. These are powerful drugs, used if the simpler medications such as beta-blockers are not proving effective.

- **Flecainide** is effective in 30 minutes, so is often used as and when the attacks have to be stopped immediately. It is a very effective medication when taken on a regular daily basis by people whose lives are made a misery by troublesome palpitations, but it is unsafe to use it at all if you have heart failure or soon after a heart attack. It can cause nausea, dizziness, and unsteady feelings. It can be used just to stop an attack, known as 'pill in the pocket' so you carry it and use it when needed.

- **Amiodarone** is a life-saving medication for some but, because of its side effects, it is not normally used as a long-term treatment unless there is no alternative. It is very effective in the management of atrial fibrillation (see below), extra beats and dangerous palpitations, and it can be used when you have heart failure and after a heart attack. It takes some time to start working and can take a long time to leave the body. Side effects include sensitivity to sunlight, skin reactions, lung problems and disturbances of the thyroid gland and liver. You will need regular supervision so that the doctor can check for side effects. Amiodarone increases the action of warfarin so extra care is needed by your doctor to monitor the blood-thinning effects of warfarin, if you are taking this.

- Other drugs less frequently used and mainly alternatives to flecainide include **disopyramide**, **propafenone** and **mexiletene**. All are effective drugs but side effects can be a problem. If you are prescribed any of these drugs, always read the package label and discuss the potential benefits and side effects with your doctor.

ATRIAL FIBRILLATION

I have just had a test for irregular heartbeats and been told that I have atrial fibrillation. What is this?

Atrial fibrillation is a very specific irregular heartbeat. The heart works like an electric circuit. There is a master switch at the top of the heart in one of the upper chambers, the atria (see Chapter 1). This switch regulates the speed of the heartbeat and normally controls how and when the heart beats, by sending messages to the muscle pump (ventricle) which is located below the atria.

When the atria fibrillate, this means that the master switch is no longer in charge, discipline is gone and chaos reigns. Atrial fibrillation occurs at around 600 beats per minute (bpm) and the top chamber (atrium) resembles a wriggling bag of worms. The heart muscle (ventricle) could therefore, in theory, be bombarded with 600 bpm and would cease to work. Fortunately below the master switch there is a junction box (called the AV node) which prevents all 600 beats getting through to the heart muscle, so the heart beats at anything up to about 180 bpm, at the rate the junction box will allow. Medication is used to further block beats through this junction box so that the rate will settle to a more normal and pleasant 70–80 bpm. Doctors refer to the fibrillation being 'poorly controlled' or 'well controlled', depending on the rate achieved after medication. Good control is when the heart beats at less than 90–100 beats per minute.

Atrial fibrillation (a fluttering feeling) is quite common and, for most people who get it, unavoidable. It responds to treatment and, although the heart is beating less efficiently than a normal regular heart rhythm, it can be improved, so that for most people it is hardly noticed. For a small number of people, it can be difficult to control and they will need to be looked after carefully.

I have been diagnosed as having atrial fibrillation. What could have caused this?

It occurs in many conditions and, in a small number of people, for no obvious reason: so-called 'lone fibrillation'. It may be a part of getting older (wear and tear to the heart) but it can be a consequence of:

- mitral valve disease;
- high blood pressure;
- coronary heart disease;
- heart failure;
- an overactive thyroid gland.

Alcohol can cause atrial fibrillation in alcoholics but can also induce it in quite normal people when they have been celebrating a little too much, particularly in women, who are more sensitive to alcohol.

How will I know that the palpitations are due to atrial fibrillation?

Atrial fibrillation may come on suddenly and fast. It is usually felt as palpitations of a rapid sort, with the heart 'beating all over the place'. It can bring on chest pain but usually makes people breathless. Naturally, it can be frightening, and may leave a feeling of light-headedness if it is so fast that the blood pressure drops a little.

Fibrillation in some people with heart failure can come and go and, as fibrillation is less efficient than normal rhythm ('sinus rhythm'), this can lead to periods of fatigue and breathlessness. For people who have atrial fibrillation regularly, it is important to keep the rate under control, or the efficiency of the heart and general well-being will be impaired.

My husband has just been told that he has atrial fibrillation. Is this dangerous and can anything be done to help him?

The short answer is: occasionally yes, it can be dangerous, but usually it is not. If he is given modern treatment, the efficiency of his heart will be improved, so that he will hardly notice that he has atrial fibrillation. If it comes on suddenly, he may become very breathless, and he may have to go into hospital. If he has an underlying heart problem, atrial fibrillation can cause little clots to form, and he will need blood thinning treatment to stop this, in order to reduce any chance of a stroke.

Tests for atrial fibrillation

My doctor has told me that I have will have to undergo some tests to check to see whether I have atrial fibrillation. What will this involve?

There are several diagnostic tests.

- Your heart may be checked by a standard resting ECG or one taken over 24 hours.
- A chest X-ray may be taken.
- A scan (echocardiogram) can be performed to check the heart valves and muscle pump (see the section *Tests* in Chapter 3).
- Blood may be taken for routine checks and to make sure that your thyroid gland is all right.

In some cases, atrial fibrillation may be part of an illness which needs surgery, such as mitral valve replacement (see Chapter 7), and

X-rays of the heart (cardiac catheterisation: see Chapter 3) will be performed before you have to undergo surgery.

You may undergo electrophysiological tests (EPS) studies (see earlier question above) if you have rapid palpitations which cannot be caught on tape, or if you have potentially dangerous palpitations and have palpitations that refuse to respond to safe and normally effective tablets. The reason for these studies is the technique of cardiac ablation (see the section *Treatment of atrial fibrillation* below).

Treatment of atrial fibrillation

What sort of treatment is there available for me now that I have been diagnosed with atrial fibrillation? Can I just be treated with medication?

Following your tests and depending on the severity of atrial fibrillation, you will usually be prescribed medication. People whose atrial fibrillation has only just started may benefit from electric shock treatment.

If you have heart problems and the fibrillation is considered part of your illness, you will be treated with medication to keep your heart rate as steady as possible. To some extent the medication used will depend on the cause.

- If you have heart failure, you may be prescribed digoxin.

- If you have high blood pressure but no muscle pump damage, you may be prescribed a beta-blocker, verapamil or diltiazam.

- Once heart failure is controlled a beta-blocker may be added to digoxin or replace it.

Most people are on a beta-blocker or verapamil (but not if they have heart failure), but some are on more than one medication to get more benefit. It is vital that you know what each type is for (write it down when you are discussing it with your doctor) because, if you stop taking one medication, your heart may race away again. You will help yourself by reducing caffeine, alcohol, stopping smoking and reducing weight.

What medication will I be offered to treat my atrial fibrillation?

Digoxin, beta-blockers (such as atenolol, bisoprolol, propranolol, metoprolol), calcium antagonists (such as verapamil, diltiazem), amiodarone, flecainide, propafenone, disopyramide, quinidine, and combinations of the above. Warfarin is used to thin your blood. See the section *Medication* in Chapter 5.

I have been told that I am going to have shock treatment for atrial fibrillation. What will this involve and is it dangerous?

If the heart is all right and it appears to have been a temporary upset, you may undergo shock treatment to get the heart back to its regular rhythm.

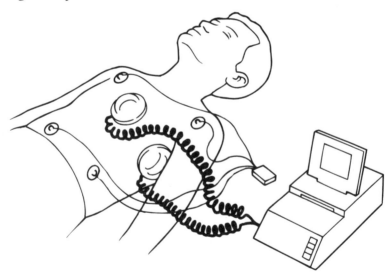

Figure 6.2 Electric shock treatment (cardioversion). Often the pad by the arm is placed on the back instead.

Electric shock treatment involves passing a high voltage electric current through your heart and is known as *cardioversion* or a DC shock. It is used to correct rhythm disturbance, such as atrial fibrillation or rapid rates from an abnormal origin, and will usually be performed if the fibrillation has been picked up early enough. The machine used is a defibrillator.

Under a brief general anaesthetic, an electric current is passed via a paddle on the top of your chest to a paddle on the left side or back (see Figure 6.2). It takes less than five minutes. The abnormal palpitation is halted at its source, and this allows the normal electrics to take over. It is successful 9 out of 10 times. Usually the patient receives warfarin for at least 4 weeks beforehand and a month afterwards to prevent the formation and dislodging of clots. If cardioversion is performed at short notice, your blood is thinned with heparin given through a vein. Cardioversion is usually done as a day-case procedure (in and out the same day) and you will notice how much better your heart behaves almost immediately.

There is no need to worry about electric shock treatment; it is safe and effective provided that all the precautions are taken – making sure of the diagnosis and use of warfarin.

A new technique involving a shock inside the heart is being used more frequently, as it appears to be more successful. A special tube is passed to the heart via the vein at the top of the leg under local anaesthetic. Once it is in place under heavy sedation or a brief general anaesthetic, a shock is delivered almost directly to the atrium, where the problem arises. The results are very encouraging, and you may be offered this as an alternative to the external shock treatment.

My cardiologist has mentioned cardiac ablation. What will this involve? Is it safe?

First, an electrophysiology study (EPS) is performed by a cardiologist in hospital (see the section *Tests* above). Once the source of the palpitation has been identified, and if the cardiologist considers you to be a suitable case, a special electrical pacemaker catheter can be placed at the source of the palpitations and radio frequency waves used to ablate them (doctors often say 'zap'!). When the cardiologist is satisfied that all is well, all catheters are removed; pressure is applied to the vein at the top of the leg for 15 minutes or so, and after two to four hours' bed rest, you will be allowed up and about; you will usually go home the next day. An ECG will be taken to check the rhythm and a 24-hour ECG may be organised to judge the effectiveness of the procedure when you are out of hospital.

Cardiac ablation can be a lengthy procedure as the catheter has to be placed very accurately. It is usually successful and abolishes the palpitations, removing or reducing the need for medication. Very rarely, the normal electrics are damaged because the abnormal electrics are very close by and they can get caught by the ablation and a pacemaker is then needed.

The procedure can remove young people from a lifetime of dependence on medication; women can become pregnant without fear of any medication damaging the baby. Also, if medication is successful but gives side effects, cardiac ablation is an effective alternative. Because ablation is a *very* individual procedure, it is important to discuss fully with your cardiologist the potential risks and the chances of benefit for you – not someone in general, but you specifically.

OTHER ABNORMAL HEARTBEATS

Two or three of my friends now have a pacemaker. Although I have 'funny' heartbeats, I have not been offered one. When are they used?

Pacemakers will be used when the heart goes too slow. The heart can alternate between fast and slow; a pacemaker will still be needed as medication given to stop the heart beating too fast will make the slowing worse. A slow heart rate is known as a *bradycardia*. When the electrics of the heart fail to connect up, this is called *heart block*.

There seem to be a lot of different methods of helping abnormal heartbeats. Why was I offered electric shock treatment and not a pacemaker?

Shock treatment corrects a rapid abnormal heartbeat whereas a pacemaker corrects a slow abnormal heartbeat. If you have a mixture of fast and slow beats, you may need both treatments. If your heart occasionally speeds up, medication may be needed in addition to a pacemaker, to stop rapid palpitations or keep them under control.

I am going to have a pacemaker fitted next month – are there different types?

There are two types that your cardiologist will choose from, depending on which is most suitable for your problem, both shown in Figure 6.3.

- A temporary pacemaker (Figure 6.3a) will be needed sometimes after a heart attack if the electrics are bruised and a block occurs – it is fitted in an emergency.

- If the electrics are permanently slower, or malfunctioning consistently, you will need a permanent pacemaker (Figures 6.3b, c). If you don't have this problem corrected, your body will lack oxygen and food; you will be tired and lethargic, and risk falling down from a blackout (see questions below). These pacemakers are small and very reliable computers which can identify your normal heartbeats and the need to fill any gaps. You may need a permanent system if your heart does not recover when the temporary system is switched off. You may be advised that one is needed when you are seen in the outpatient clinic, because your heart has been found to go too slowly at times.

I am rather nervous about having a pacemaker fitted. What will it involve?

For a permanent system, you will usually stay one night in hospital, although your hospital may undertake to fit the pacemaker as a day case. You will be told how long your stay is likely to be so that you can prepare a night bag if necessary.

For a *temporary* pacemaker, a wire is passed via a vein in the arm, neck or below your collarbone (most often) to the right ventricle (pumping chamber) and connected to a box at the bedside or attached to your arm (see Figure 6.3a). It is fitted under local anaesthesia. This senses normal beats and fills any gaps with pacemaker beats. When the electrics recover, it is removed by simply pulling the wire out; this is not painful.

For a *permanent* pacemaker, you will be given a local anaesthetic and sedation; then one or two wires are passed to your heart via a vein under the collarbone (the subclavian vein), or the one running on the inside of your shoulder (cephalic vein). The pacemaker box is attached and buried under the skin. The wires are positioned with X-ray guidance and the procedure takes about one hour. A small cut is needed on the front of your chest below the collarbone and stitches will be used to close it up at the end of the procedure. Stitches that do not dissolve will be removed 7 to 10 days later, usually by the nurse at your doctor's surgery. Before you leave hospital, a chest X-ray will check that all is well, and the technician will use a computer placed on the skin over the pacemaker box to make sure that it is working properly.

Before my heart started to play up, I was very active. Will I be able to go back to that sort of activity when I have had my pacemaker inserted?

The short answer is yes. A pacemaker is all about correcting a problem and allowing you to lead a normal active life. You will need the stitches out a week after the insertion and you will have been

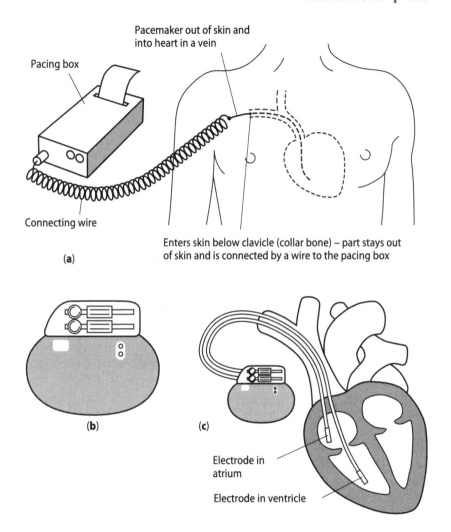

Figure 6.3 Pacemakers.
(**a**) Temporary pacemaker;
(**b**) Permanent pacemaker;
(**c**) Permanent pacemaker in position.

given a course of antibiotics to protect you from infection. You will not be allowed to drive a car for a week, and you must inform the DVLA and your car insurance company. You may be able to hold a Group II licence if there are no other disqualifying conditions, but you will need to wait 6 weeks. Group I licences are for motorcyclists, car and light goods vehicle drivers; group II relates to drivers of vehicles in excess of 3.5 metric tonnes laden weight, and bus or coach drivers. Group II standards apply to emergency police, firemen, ambulance drivers and taxi drivers.

You will be given a check of your pacemaker function at 1 month and then once a year. This yearly check is to monitor its battery life. If the batteries begin to run down (many last over 10 years), the box will be unplugged from the wires and a new box implanted under sedation and local anaesthetic.

You will be given a card to carry with you at all times. You will need to tell airport security as you will set off the alarms. Modern household microwaves and electricity do not affect it but mobile phones may do if placed close to the box (about 10 cm). Avoid placing them in shirt or jacket pockets on the pacemaker side. You will not be able to have an magnetic resonance imaging scan.

Life should not be restricted just because of a pacemaker.

Can pacemakers be troublesome?

Not usually, but occasionally they can cause soreness and, very rarely, become infected (it will then need to be removed). They may need adjusting from time to time – this is done via a computer placed over the box on the outside of the skin. Some early pacemakers developed faults and needed replacing. The wires in the heart do not usually displace after the first 24–48 hours. You can damage the wire or box in a heavy fall or accident, and it should be checked if this happens. Contact sports such as soccer or rugby should be avoided. Most people have no problems at all but, if you do have concerns, contact your pacemaker clinic for advice.

When I went to see the cardiologist, he was very frank with me and said that the type of heart rhythm that I had was rather dangerous. He wants to insert an implantable defibrillator. Is this a type of pacemaker?

The official name for this is an *automatic implantable cardioverter defibrillator* or AICD and, yes, it also acts as a pacemaker.

Some people have a very dangerous rhythm tendency which could cause them to drop dead suddenly. For people like you pacemaker wires are passed into the heart, under general or local anaesthetic, through the top of your chest wall through a big vein which runs under your collarbone (*subclavian*). The defibrillator box is attached and then buried under the skin of your chest wall; sometimes it is placed in the abdomen in your stomach area. It recognises normal beats but, if abnormal dangerous beats occur, it shocks your heart immediately. This may be felt as a slight thump. The machine needs checking at regular intervals to make sure that the battery life is satisfactory and, because it is a type of computer, it can also keep a check on how often it has been used. It is an expensive option but a definite lifesaver.

The British Heart Foundation book *Implantable cardioverter defibrillators* is a superb guide for patient and family (see Appendix 3).

A friend of mine has a defibrillator for atrial fibrillation – is this a new treatment?

Atrial defibrillators are rarely used. They are used in people who get very occasional attacks of atrial fibrillation – say, two or three a year. They are inserted under local anaesthetic similar to a pacemaker, and provide a shock to correct the atrial fibrillation when an attack occurs.

BLACKOUTS

My wife has suffered from blackouts recently. Can you tell me what these are and what causes them?

A blackout is a sudden loss of consciousness; this causes her to fall to the floor. If your wife's heart suddenly goes too fast or too slow, her blood pressure falls and she will collapse. It happens very suddenly; her colour drains away ('as white as a sheet'), but recovery is usually quick. You will probably notice that your wife's skin becomes flushed. Often she will recover so quickly that she may think that she has tripped up and 'wonder what the fuss was about'.

Sometimes it may be a faint, but blackouts can also be caused by lack of blood (anaemia), and problems with the nervous system (the brain), and a low blood sugar, for example in epilepsy or lack of blood from narrowed arteries. Blackouts from a heart problem tend to be sudden in onset with a quick recovery (5–10 minutes); blackouts *not* caused by a heart problem may be sudden in onset but recovery is slow, sometimes over several hours.

My wife has been ignoring these blackouts because they don't happen too often. Should I get her to go to the doctor and have them investigated?

Yes, or she could fall and injure herself. Your wife may need a pacemaker or medication to keep them under control.

How does a faint differ from a blackout?

Before a faint there is usually a warning. You may become pale and sweaty, yawn a lot and have a buzzing in your ears. Faints often occur in a warm, close environment or when you have been standing for a long time in heat or a queue. A bad coughing bout can bring on a faint (*cough syncope*) and it can occur if men (and rarely women) get up suddenly at night to pass urine (*micturition syncope*). *Syncope* (pronounced 'sin-co-pee') is the medical word for a sudden loss of consciousness.

If my wife feels faint, what should I do to help?

Help her to lie down flat and raise her legs. As she recovers, gradually get her into the sitting position and then let her stand up. Make sure she is steady on her feet before she walks again.

7 | Valve disease

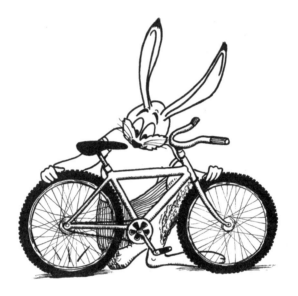

This book is primarily about heart health and coronary artery disease. Sometimes heart valves become diseased, so a brief account of valve problems and their treatment is provided here.

The heart contains four valves which are designed to make sure that the blood flows one way only (see Figure 1.2 on p. 6). Disease of the valves will distort the normal function of the heart. The two valves that are the most important are the mitral and aortic valves and these are the most commonly affected (see Chapter 1 for information on anatomy). Sometimes both can be affected at the same time. Each year 5000 people in the UK have valve surgery.

Two disorders can sometimes affect the aortic and mitral valves:

- they can leak (this is called *incompetence*);

- they can narrow (this is called *stenosis*).

The aortic valve normally has three flaps (leaflets) but some people are born with two and this causes early wear and tear. The normal three-leaflet valve may also harden up or become leaky with age. This can occur independently of coronary artery disease.

CAUSES

I have been diagnosed with valve disease. What do you think is likely to have caused it?

There are several causes of valve disease.

- **Mitral stenosis** (narrowing) can be caused by rheumatic fever. This condition, usually experienced in childhood or teens, can inflame the valves and lining of the heart, leaving permanent damage.

- **Mitral incompetence** (leaking) may be the result of rheumatic fever, bacterial infection (see below), a weakness of the valve supports causing the leaflets to flop backwards, or a narrowing of the coronary arteries.

- **Aortic stenosis** may be due to rheumatic fever, being born with an abnormal valve (congenital) or age (wear and tear).

- **Aortic incompetence** may be due to rheumatic fever, high blood pressure, bacterial infection, age, or being born with an abnormal valve.

SYMPTOMS

How will I recognise valvular disease?

If the aortic valve narrows, this can cause angina, breathlessness and blackouts, whereas, if it leaks, it usually causes the heart to enlarge and breathlessness then follows. If you feel tired and breathless on exertion, it is probably a good idea to go to the doctor for an opinion or tests. Valve disease may cause heart failure (see Chapter 5).

A severe mitral valve leak or narrowing will also cause breathlessness.

Both valves can become infected (see the section *Infection* below).

Does the fact that I have valve disease mean that there is a greater strain on my heart?

Yes. As a result of either narrowing or leaking, or both, the abnormal valves increase the work that the heart has to do. If the valve is narrowed, the pump must generate higher and higher pressures to get the blood through. If the valve leaks, the pump must put out more blood with each beat: it must pump out the 5 litres that the body needs each minute plus the volume that has leaked back.

TESTS

I have been asked to go for tests to see if I have valve disease. What will these involve?

The doctor can usually hear heart murmurs and will confirm the diagnosis with echocardiography (see Chapter 5). Sometimes a murmur is heard and a problem detected by chance. The echocardiogram provides a comprehensive picture of your heart, telling us about any valve leaks or narrowing and their severity. If your valve condition is not too bad, it can be watched by the echocardiogram at 12- or 6-monthly intervals. If the echo identifies a severe problem, you will be offered further investigations and possible surgery.

TREATMENT

Valve conditions that are not severe can initially be treated medically. Diuretics (water tablets: see Chapter 2) are used to relieve breathlessness; digoxin may be used if there is atrial fibrillation (Chapter 6), when warfarin will also be used. If the main problem is a leaky valve, ACE inhibitors (see Chapter 2) may be used to try to reduce the leak. They act to open up the arteries so that blood leaving the heart meets less resistance, with the idea being to make it easier for blood to flow forwards rather than leak backwards.

I have had tests for valve disease and have been put on a waiting list for a new valve. It all sounds rather frightening –what will this involve?

Valve surgery is routine for the surgeon but a daunting experience for anyone about to undergo it! The surgeon should discuss with you the risks to you individually (if he doesn't, ask him) and explain what sort of valves are available and what the options are.

Preparation is similar to that for a coronary bypass operation (see Chapter 2). Your breast bone (*sternum*) will be cut along its length and your heart stopped; you will then be put on a bypass machine while your heart is being operated on. The surgeon will open up your heart to get access to the valves as these are located inside the heart. Sometimes a leaking mitral valve can be repaired and surgeons will do this if at all possible. Otherwise, an artificial valve is put in after the diseased valve has been cut out.

Your hospital stay will usually be 7–10 days. All heart surgery is a 'big operation' but we are lucky these days to have perfected the techniques and the risks are therefore minimised.

What are artificial heart valves like?

There are two sorts of valves used – tissue valves and mechanical valves. The decision as to which sort of valve to use will be made by the surgeon at the time of the operation, because it's only then that a considered decision can be made. The surgeon will have explained the differences to you beforehand, and you can indicate your preference should the surgeon have a choice when the operation is being performed.

- **Tissue valves** are made of natural tissue from humans, cows or pigs. They are treated to avoid rejection later.

- **Mechanical valves** are usually made of carbon fibre (but are often called metal or plastic valves) and contain no natural tissue. They may click.

A big difference between the two types is the need for warfarin, needed for ever if you receive a mechanical valve, whereas aspirin is all that will be needed if a tissue type is used (unless you are in atrial fibrillation).

How long do these different types of valve last?

Mechanical valves last many years and rarely go wrong. Tissue valves can wear out after 10 years but the more modern ones last longer. Tissue valves are easier to live with but the chances of needing a repeat operation are higher.

It sounds like a big operation. What are my chances of pulling through?

Survival after a single valve replacement is 96%. There may be a slightly increased risk if coronary surgery is needed at the same time. This is more likely in older patients. Without an operation to replace a severely diseased valve, few people live beyond 2 years and quality of life is poor with a relentless downhill slide. Valve surgery will offer you an excellent chance of being alive and well 10 years on.

What happens if something goes wrong later? Can valve operations be repeated?

Yes. Repeat operations are generally safe to do and about 10% (one in ten) tissue valves need redoing after 10–15 years.

Do all diseased valves need an operation?

No, many minor problems never cause any concern. However, you will be checked regularly just in case these problems worsen. Even badly damaged valves need not be operated on straight away; the cardiologist will keep an eye on your condition and action will only being taken when symptoms become a problem.

Are there any other types of surgery for valve disease? I have been told there is something called 'balloon surgery'. What is this?

Leaking valves will need surgery. A narrow mitral valve, however, can be widened with a balloon. The decision to use a balloon depends on what is found when you have transoesophageal echocardiography (see Chapter 3). If your case is suitable, a balloon operation on the mitral valve (*mitral valvuloplasty*) will be as successful as surgery.

Mitral valvuloplasty takes place in the cardiac catheter laboratory with a technique similar to coronary angioplasty (see Chapter 3).

Under local anaesthetic, the vein at the top of the leg is used. The vein goes into the right atrium which is separated from the left atrium by the atrial septum (see Chapter 1). The mitral valve lies between the left atrium and left ventricle, so the balloon needs to be in the left atrium in order to find its way through the valve. The septum is in the way, so a small hole is made in the atrial septum with a special needle which allows the cardiologist to position a large balloon behind and then through the valve. This method is necessary as the valve opens away from the cardiologist allowing the balloon to be passed forwards into the opening – the cardiologist more or less floats the balloon through as the valve opens with the blood flow. The balloon is blown up in the valve which is then split open along the flaps that have become stuck together. When the balloon and tubes are removed, the cardiologist will press on your groin over the vein to stop the bleeding. No stitches are used. If there are no complications, you will go home the next day.

If you can balloon a narrow valve without heart surgery, can you replace valves also?

Recently, techniques have been developed in very specialised centres to repair a leaking mitral valve and replace the aortic valve, using access from the vein or artery in the groin. It is very early days and these procedures are mainly used in people who are unfit for conventional heart surgery.

INFECTION

I am about to undergo valve surgery. Are there any problems associated with valve replacement?

Heart valves can become infected and this is known as *bacterial endocarditis* (pronounced 'en-doe-car-dye-tiss'). It can affect replacement valves and your own valves if they are diseased. Infection is not common but it is preventable. Your teeth and gums must be kept healthy: regular dental check-ups are needed. Bugs can enter the bloodstream via tooth decay while you are chewing. If you are considered a high risk case, any operative procedure that you undergo should be covered by a course of antibiotics to protect the valves – the medical term for this is *antibiotic prophylaxis*. Special antibiotic preparations are available on prescription. Check with your doctor.

Though rare, an infection that damages a valve is very dangerous and only half of infected people survive. As infection is preventable, this is one of those times when prevention really is life-saving. Recently the National Institute for Clinical Excellence (NICE) has declined to recommended antibiotic prophylaxis for people at increased risk of endocarditis when they undergo dental procedures, but emphasised the importance of maintaining good oral health.

I had a valve replacement some months ago. How will I know if I have developed an infection?

Infections develop slowly but you will increasingly notice these symptoms:

- raised temperature;
- sweating at night time;
- feeling more and more ill;
- weight loss;
- poor appetite;
- joint aches and pains.

If you develop any of these symptoms, go straight to your doctor. If the doctor suspects endocarditis, he will send you directly to hospital.

When I was in hospital for a valve replacement, one of the patients there had developed an infection. Is infection common? Is it likely that I shall develop an infection too?

It is not common, but it is preventable. Apart from maintaining oral health, you should avoid tattooing and body piercing. If it is caught early, 50% of people will recover. Therefore, you should always be aware of the possible problems and symptoms. If you develop any of the symptoms discussed above, go straight to your doctor. You can get a credit card-sized warning card from the British Heart Foundation (see Appendix 2).

8 | Sex and the heart

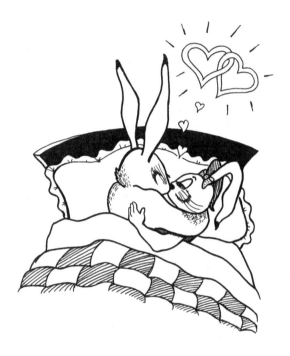

Having heart disease does not mean the end of an enjoyable, satisfying sex life.

For anyone who was previously sexually active, failing to resume sexual enjoyment may cause unnecessary frustration, irritability and marital discord. This applies to men and women in heterosexual relationships and the gay community. It is a long-standing stable sexual relationship that is important and, if it existed before the heart problem was detected, it should continue afterwards. Casual sex may be more stressful to your heart and this is discussed in a question below.

A new relationship developing after heart disease that has been diagnosed in one or both partners should not present problems providing it has none of the dangers of a casual encounter. Relationships based on trust, understanding and love are not casual, and as they develop, no undue stress is placed on the heart. Above all else, if you are involved in a loving new relationship, do not let your anatomical heart interfere with your emotional and happy heart!

QUESTIONS YOU MAY FIND DIFFICULT TO ASK YOUR DOCTOR

What happens to my heart when I am making love?

As you become aroused, your heart rate begins to increase and you breathe a little faster; as the excitement increases, both the heart rate and the blood pressure increase, reaching their peak at orgasm and settling back to resting levels after about three minutes' rest. The average duration of sex is 15 minutes and the heart is really only stressed for 3 minutes.

If the heart rate is increasing, is sex stressful to the heart?

Sex is just another form of exercise as far as the heart is concerned. We have already said (in Chapter 3) that angina pain can be brought on by exercise, so pain could occur during sex, but the important point is that sexual activity is no more stressful to the heart than other normal daily activities. In one study using tape recordings of the heart beats during sex, the heart rate averaged 120 beats per minute and was less than that often seen during other daily activities. In another study, the blood pressure rise was not found to be dangerous or exaggerated.

The stress to the heart during sex is the same as 4 minutes on a treadmill exercise ECG. If you can do more than 4 minutes on that, making love should be OK. If your partner needs to be reassured, ask the doctor to arrange for the exercise ECG test to be performed in the presence of your partner.

Is casual sex more stressful to the heart than with a partner in a long-term relationship?

Yes, casual sex can be more stressful. Long-standing relationships, where people are comfortable with each other, should present no problem, but a casual encounter can lead to a greater heart rate rise. This is not harmful to a normal heart, but if coronary disease is present, problems may occur. There may be an age mis-match (older man, younger woman) and the environment unfamiliar (a hotel room), following too much food and drink (casual sex at an office party). 'Playing away' can therefore be risky.

You sometimes hear horror stories of people dying while they are making love. Are these stories true?

You can die at any time and this includes during sex! The risk during sex is very low indeed and no higher than during other normal daily activities. However, it may be significant that, of those who die or have a heart attack during sex, 75% are having extra-marital sex, and 95% are men: so the advice is, beware!

I had a heart attack recently. How soon can I start making love again?

After a heart attack, providing there were no complications, sexual activity can be resumed in 2–3 weeks. Ask your doctor and use a stairs, walking or treadmill test (see below) as your guide. The advice is the same whether the patient is male or female.

Sex is normal and not unduly stressful for couples with a long-standing relationship and should be enjoyed as much by those with heart disease as those without. As you recover from a heart attack and return to normal activities, you should be able to return to the normal activity of sex.

I am in my early fifties and have had a heart attack. Am I too old for sex?

Age is not a barrier and even those in their seventies or eighties, who were previously sexually active, should not be afraid of resuming normal relations.

Men may take longer getting an erection and women may worry they are less attractive and find vaginal lubrication a problem (see question below on K-Y jelly). Sex should not be rushed – we have road rage but we don't need sex rage! Take your time, enjoy the build-up and use lubricants if necessary. Age is a time for mature reflection, and a few wrinkles here and there do not detract from the beauty of the person within.

I had heart surgery 3 weeks ago. My husband is keen to make love again. Can I resume lovemaking safely?

You can resume as soon as you feel able. Chest wall pain can be a problem particularly when you are positioned underneath your husband. Mutual foreplay without full sex can be a satisfying alternative and may be a good way to restart sexual activity, particularly if your chest wall gives you some pain. Alternatively, try the side-to-side position, or experiment to find a position that is comfortable to both of you (see below).

After angioplasty, you can resume sex within two to three days, depending on whether your groin is bruised or painful.

As a useful guide, the stress on the heart equates to walking briskly (in 10 seconds) up and down two flights of household stairs (13 steps each) or walking one mile on the flat in 20 minutes. If no pain or undue breathlessness occurs, then sex should be symptom free. If angina does occur during one of these tests, repeat it following sublingual nitrate tablets or spray. If nitrates are effective, they can be taken before sex. Indeed, as a side effect, there is some evidence that nitrates improve sexual pleasure. Nitrates should not be used if Viagra, Levitra or Cialis has been taken.

My partner has recently had heart surgery but has been given
the all clear. Are some positions during lovemaking dangerous?

No, not within the bounds of common sense. The heart does not
appear to be unduly stressed in any position as long as the
relationship is long-standing. Casual sex can be more stressful to the
heart (see question above). See the question below about different
positions that may be helpful.

The coarse hair which grows back on your partner's chest, where
it has been shaved, may be uncomfortable for you ('it feels like a
hedgehog'), and a small soft cushion placed between you can help (the
sort of size you get on aeroplanes).

Since I came back from hospital following a heart attack, I've
had no interest in making love. It upsets my partner and
frustrates him. What should I say to him?

Most people resume sex as frequently as before the heart attack or
surgery but others are less active. Some people are afraid that
sex may damage the heart, spoiling a previously enjoyable sex life.
They are often influenced by what is called 'Hollywood sex', which is
the movie portrayal of overenthusiastic sex; in real life, sex may not be
such a grand performance, and the stress on the heart is therefore not
exaggerated.

Anxiety and depression may decrease your desire but, as your
condition improves, your desire usually returns. Because you have a
heart problem, you are now more aware of the heart beating, whereas
before it had never concerned you. It will increase during lovemaking
but there is nothing to fear: do the stair or walking test again to
reassure yourself (see above).

If you are depressed (which is not unusual) after your heart attack
or surgery, it usually lifts quickly (90% of the time), but a small
number of people will continue to feel depressed and this will reduce
or remove any desire for sex. When you do make love (infrequently),
it is not fulfilling. Do not accept this situation – you are not 'past it' –

seek help from your doctor. Medication for depression – often for only a short time – is very effective and side effects are not usually a problem.

At first, it may be that just touching, holding and caressing without intercourse will help you slowly return to a full sex life.

I have been diagnosed with angina. Will heart disease affect my sex drive?

No. There are too many people who believe in myths like this. Some think that their sex life is all over when they get to 50. This should be the prime of life. In medical terms, you will be pleased to know that middle age extends to 70 years! Once your symptoms have been dealt with, you should be able to resume lovemaking.

My wife and I have always had a vigorous and adventurous love life. Now I am worried that I may get angina while I am making love. Is this likely?

Angina may occur and is best treated with sublingual nitrates beforehand. Keep nitrates by the bedside, and take an extra spray or tablet if angina occurs during sex. Rest for 5–10 minutes, then resume if you wish to. If prolonged pain occurs, it could be a heart attack (this is very unusual): if the pain persists after 30 minutes, seek medical help. If angina is of a severity to limit sexual activity on a regular basis, you should be considered for fuller investigation with a view to angioplasty or surgery.

Breathlessness during sex may respond to nitrates but, if heart failure is the problem, your partner will need to adopt a more active role, and different positions could be tried. If you don't usually lie underneath, try this less stressful position or sit in a chair with your partner astride, facing you.

To be honest, our love life wasn't up to much before the heart attack. Will it get worse?

If you were having sexual difficulties (such as lack of interest, poor satisfaction, or inability to sustain or develop an erection if you are male) before your heart problems, these will get worse. It is important to talk about these problems, either individually or together with the doctor or members of the rehabilitation team. Specific sexual counselling from trained counsellors may help.

I have heart failure and find that sex is too much effort. What can I do?

This is difficult because your heart's pumping action has been reduced. The ACE inhibitors or AII antagonists improve the heart's output and may help (see Chapter 2). Ask your doctor about them if you have not been prescribed them. Water pills (diuretics) may cause erectile dysfunction (impotence) as a side effect but you should not stop taking these.

It may be possible to reduce the dosage which can help. Unfortunately, if your breathing depends on taking diuretics, the dosage will not be reduced.

Heart failure patients may be unable to sustain a full sexual relationship but cuddling, caressing, close contact and even foreplay will still enable you to enjoy a satisfying relationship.

Let your partner do most of the physical work and try different positions. If you are male and find that you can't get an erection, ask about available treatments (see next questions).

I am taking medication for my heart problem. Can medication affect my sex life?

The most obvious side effect of medication is male impotence – now known as erectile dysfunction or ED. Sometimes sex drive or desire (known as *libido*) can be reduced. Women may experience problems with arousal, desire, orgasm or feel pain due to lubrication problems. Drugs can be a problem, but it is most often the condition itself that leads to the ED in men. If a prescribed drug causes sexual problems it will do so in the first 2–4 weeks of its use and an alternative would then be worth trying. The drugs most often linked to ED are the beta-blockers and diuretics. and in the female, sex drive or interest can be affected by beta-blockers. Statins used to lower cholesterol also very rarely cause sexual difficulties – mainly ED in the male.

Whilst these effects may be drug-induced, they may also be psychological or due to your heart problem itself. Whatever you do, don't stop your medication, as this may lead to more heart problems; equally, don't accept the situation. Talk to your doctor: this is not a time to be shy or 'British'. Ask your doctor whether the tablets might affect your sex life. The doctor will know what you are talking about. Changing medication or adjusting dosage may help. If you are feeling depressed, antidepressants may correct the problem. However, if ED or sexual dysfunction (such as poor female lubrication or lack of interest) continues, it should be evaluated further. You may be given hormones, and men may have their prostate checked. Get specialist advice.

Since being on blood pressure pills, my husband is having a problem getting an erection. Is there a connection?

Yes. Blood pressure tablets can sometimes cause erection failure in men and may affect some women also. If this happens, your husband should tell his doctor because a change in medication could solve the problem. Erectile dysfunction is more common with diuretics and beta-blockers and less likely with angiotensin II antagonists and doxazosin.

Everyone has heard about Viagra. My husband has a poor erection: will it help him?

Viagra is a truly wonderful drug, but it does not suit or help everyone with erection problems (known as erectile dysfunction or ED). In 8 out of 10 people it helps restore an erection in men. It is not an aphrodisiac, so the penis will still need normal stimulation to make Viagra work. Doses are 25, 50 and 100 mg, taken 1 hour before sexual foreplay, and its effects lasts for 4–6 hours. Heart patients may benefit from Viagra because heart disease, rather than the drugs used to treat it, is the most common cause of ED. Always get advice from your doctor and do not buy it on the Internet. It does not cause heart attacks (nor do other treatments), any more than might occur by chance. Before trying it, you should have a check-up at the doctor's, and you may be asked to do an exercise ECG. Viagra reacts with nitrates and nicorandil (see the section *Treatment* in Chapter 3). Oral nitrates and nicorandil must be stopped for 1 week before Viagra is used, and the nitrate tablets under the tongue or spray should not be used for 12 hours before or after Viagra. Nitrates plus Viagra can cause a dangerous fall in blood pressure. Otherwise, Viagra is a very safe and effective treatment, providing you are guided medically – do not experiment without a medical opinion.

A friend of mine had a heart attack after taking Viagra: it seems dangerous to me. What do media reports say?

There is no increased risk of a heart attack from Viagra – in fact there were fewer cases when Viagra was compared with a placebo (where there was no active tablet taken). Your friend probably took it without medical advice.

Does the effect of Viagra wear off the more you use it?

No. After a year, 87 out of 100 men who benefited from it, still did so.

What happens if I get angina during sex after taking Viagra?

Do not use a nitrate tablet or spray at the same time. Stop your activity and sit or stand up. The pain should gradually settle. A glass of whisky or brandy might be helpful. Do not try again until you have discussed the event with your doctor.

Are there other heart drugs that may react with Viagra?

Currently you are advised not to be on nicorandil (a potassium channel activator) or nevibolol (a beta-blocker) until research has reported that it is safe to do so.

Nitrates help my angina but I would like to try Viagra – what should I do?

Nitrates are relatively weak angina drugs, and have no proven benefit in preventing heart attacks or sudden death. They are used only to help relieve pain and breathlessness. Alternatives exist, so you can ask for your medicine to be changed. For example, you could try felodipine or amlodipine as alternatives. Once the change has proved successful (two weeks should be enough time), you can then try Viagra. Your doctor may need to ask a specialist about this, but most people can manage without nitrates.

I have tried Viagra but it only partly works – how can I improve things?

First of all don't despair. Viagra does not always work first time you try it – indeed some people need seven or eight attempts before it 'kicks in'. If it is not effective at 50 mg, try the 100 mg tablet. Only one tablet a day is advised and it should be taken on an empty stomach, and no smoking or alcohol is advised. It begins to work in 30 minutes, is at its peak after 1 hour and gives you 'a window of opportunity' for 4–6 hours. Remember that you have to be stimulated for it to work. Side effects are not common. Headache and flushing with occasional indigestion occur but are not usually severe enough to warrant stopping taking it.

I have heard of newer Viagra-like drugs – are they any different?

There are two drugs that work the same way as Viagra – Levitra and Cialis. Their real names are sildenafil (Viagra), vardenafil (Levitra) and tadalafil (Cialis). They all work in the same way, by blocking an enzyme known as phosphodiesterase-5 (PDE5) which controls blood flow to the penis. Blocking PDE5 increases flow, so an erection occurs.

Levitra is very like Viagra and works at 5, 10 or 20 mg and, like Viagra, it is best to take it on an empty stomach to get the full effect by 1 hour. However, sex with a full stomach is not a good idea for heart patients. It is as effective as Viagra, so we can say it is an alternative which is worth trying.

Cialis is different in one way – it lasts longer. It is available as 10 or 20 mg equal to 50 or 100 mg of Viagra. It reaches its peak effect 1–2 hours after it is taken but may be active 36 hours later. It is not affected by food. Side effects are similar for all three drugs but muscle pains are more common with Cialis. ED success rates are similar. Cialis may, for some, allow more spontaneity but nitrates or nicorandil cannot be used for 48 hours afterwards. If you think you can't have sex without the risk of angina, Viagra's shorter action will be better for you, but when your condition has been stabilised and well controlled you will probably be given the choice.

Studies have confirmed the safety of all three drugs but they should only be obtained after advice from a healthcare professional and from reputable sources. Daily therapy with Cialis has now been approved at 2.5 and 5 mg doses which may allow more regular and spontaneous sex. You can use all three drugs if you want – for example, Cialis on Friday evening for a romantic weekend and Viagra as Levitra when a quicker action is needed. Many men like to try all three as there are slight differences and personal preferences are different; also, the hardness of the erection may vary.

If tablets don't work do I have any other choices?

Indeed you do, so do not give up in despair. No treatment for ED harms the heart, so if one is safe, so are the others. Injection therapy and vacuum pumps are highly effective but need specialised advice, so ask for a referral. Before giving up on the Viagra approach, make sure you have tried the top dose. If you cannot take Viagra because you are on nitrates or nicorandil and they cannot be stopped, then there are other choices available (see next questions).

Can I mix medications?

You can, but there is no safety information or clear research evidence of benefit. It is not recommended outside carefully controlled research studies.

All I hear about is men's problems – do women get sexual difficulties and can they be helped, with Viagra for example?

Women certainly have sexual difficulties – known as female sexual dysfunction or FSD. Research is being done to see if treatments will help. The real problem is that the problem in men with getting an erection is obvious, whereas women's problems are not. Most doctors are men and have not been asking the right questions! Lubrication after the menopause is discussed above. Some drugs appear to suppress libido (sex drive or interest) and affect orgasms. Heart disease may also affect sexual confidence, as well as be a cause of reducing sexual enjoyment. Viagra may help, but we lack proof, so it is currently not recommended for women. Guidance is not really very clear, but still mention any problems that you are having – although we do not have clear-cut recommendations, by applying basic medicine and common sense, we may be able to help. Unless women raise the problem, the medical profession will not be aware of its scale and progress will be slow in helping.

Can you give me some advice in preparing for sex since my heart attack?

When heart disease has been diagnosed, it is important to follow the lifestyle changes discussed in previous chapters, and particularly in Chapters 9 and 10. Improving exercise ability and losing weight will help sexual ability also. Here is some practical advice to minimise the stress on the heart during sex.

- Avoid sex within two hours of a bath or a heavy meal. Taking a shower and eating a light salad will be better.

- Keep the bedroom and sheets warm. You could invest in an electric blanket if it is cold.

- Don't make love if you are tired at the end of the day. Wait until the morning when you are refreshed and relaxed.

- Avoid caffeine, smoking or alcohol before or after sex. Alcohol may raise expectations that you cannot fulfil and it certainly does not enhance your sex life!

- If you get angina, use your nitrate tablets before lovemaking (but not if you are using Viagra, Levitra or Cialis).

- Don't rush into it – take your time.

- Use lubricants if necessary (see question below).

I have heard that K-Y jelly can be useful if lovemaking is a problem or painful. How safe is it to use?

K-Y jelly is a lubricant which can be particularly useful if your vagina is dry. This sometimes occurs after the menopause and can be a problem in patients with heart problems who naturally, but unnecessarily, feel reluctant or are afraid of resuming a normal sex life. K-Y jelly has no effect on the heart and is totally safe. It does not reduce the effectiveness of condoms or damage them. Topical oestrogens are also effective, and other non-hormonal moisturisers are available.

Where anal intercourse is practised, K-Y jelly is very helpful at reducing any physical trauma to the anus or penis, the pain of which occasionally causes palpitations (see question below).

Does oral or anal sex stress the heart?

Oral sex should not stress your heart, providing both you and your partner are comfortable with it.

There is some evidence that anal sex increases palpitations but this has not been proved in a secure long-standing homosexual relationship.

I have resumed sex after my bypass and there are no problems, but I'm afraid that it might do some damage to the operation site. Is this possible?

Firstly, it is good to know that you have returned to a normal sexual relationship – we would like all people undergoing heart surgery such as yours to achieve the same, because it is safe and enjoyable. To answer your question directly – no, the operation cannot be damaged: stitches will not be torn and nothing will fall apart! It is important to remember that sex should be an enjoyable fulfilling experience whether there is heart disease or not – people with heart disease can enjoy a sexual relationship whatever their age.

I read in the newspaper that ED could be a marker for silent coronary disease. Is this true?

Yes. Over 50% of men with coronary disease have some degree of erectile dysfunction (ED) and it can occur 2–5 years before a coronary event. This is why men with ED and no heart complaints need checking for silent heart disease: their lives may depend on it.

My husband has lost all interest in sex even though he has made a good recovery from his small heart attack. Is it my fault?

Loss of interest in sex is known as loss of libido. It is not something you should blame yourself for. It could be a result of ED – a kind of vicious circle. A low testosterone level leads to lack of sex drive and sometimes ED. Your husband should be checked by his family doctor and get a blood test (before 10 a.m.) for testosterone.

Men with low testosterones are more likely to get coronary disease but we don't know if replacing or boosting it prevents coronary disease. If his testosterone is low, replacing it with a topical gel daily or an injection every 8–10 weeks can make the world of difference, restoring libido and overall energy and well-being. Tests for prostate cancer (prostate specific antigen, PSA) are done on the same blood sample because of a (very controversial) possible link between testosterone and prostate cancer – this is a precaution and should not put anyone off getting tested. As men get older, testosterone gradually falls but replacement or boosting works at all ages. No man or woman should consider themselves 'too old' for intimacy.

9 | Diet

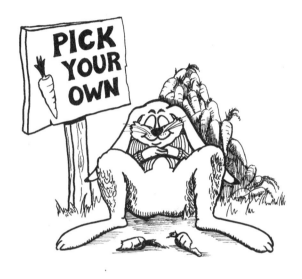

There has been a lot of talk about diet, both in this book and in the media in general, about the importance of good, healthy eating to keep your heart in good shape. The questions below will answer, I hope, all the questions that you may have about food types, a healthy diet and losing weight. When we use the word 'diet' we do not mean crash diets to lose weight, but adopting a healthy lifestyle with balanced nutrition, which is far more important and safer.

In the past, many doctors have doubted the importance of lowering cholesterol, and have in many ways hindered the management and prevention of coronary artery disease. We now have overwhelming evidence that a high cholesterol causes coronary disease, and that lowering it encourages heart health and prevents the consequences of coronary disease by reducing heart attacks and the need for surgery or angioplasty. Fears that lowering cholesterol simply meant that you died just as soon but from something else have been totally disproved and the evidence accumulates daily to support the view that not only do people have less heart disease but they live better lives for longer. If you stop smoking, you will reduce your chances of lung cancer and heart disease; if you reduce your cholesterol you will reduce your chances of heart disease and stroke.

Eating healthily does not mean a boring diet. As the British Heart Foundation puts it 'Food should be fun' and can be healthy too. It's all about avoiding a premature death.

FOOD TYPES AND EATING HEALTHILY

Fats

Fats or lipids are discussed fully in Chapter 2 in the section *Risks of high cholesterol levels*. We discuss here what types of food are involved. Remember that fats are divided into saturated and unsaturated types and most foods contain a combination. The proportion varies depending on the food chosen.

Saturated fats are mainly of animal origin. They are usually hard at room temperature. They can also be found in some vegetable fats. Too much saturated fat can be bad for the heart and it is the saturated fat that raises cholesterol. They are found in:

- red meat;
- butter, milk, cheese, cream;
- suet and lard;
- some vegetable fats, especially coconut and palm oil;
- cakes, biscuits;

- chocolate; and

- most puddings.

Unsaturated fats are mainly of vegetable origin. They are liquid or soft solids at room temperature. There are two types:

- *polyunsaturated*, found in sunflower oil, soft margarines labelled 'high in polyunsaturates'; these fats can lower cholesterol;

- *monounsaturates*, found in olive and rapeseed oil.

Table 9.1 Content of omega-3 polyunsaturated fatty acids in oily fish

Oily fish	Omega-3 content (g per 100g)
Mackerel	2.2
Herring	1.7
Sardines	1.7
Pilchards	1.7
Lake trout	1.6
Salmon	1.4
Halibut	0.9
Rainbow trout	0.6
Tuna (less if tinned)	0.5

I have read that fish oil is very good for you. Can you tell me about this?

Oily fish contain a particular type of polyunsaturated fat (omega-3 fatty acid) and this has been shown to help prevent coronary disease partly by thinning the blood. Table 9.1 shows the healthiest fish to eat.

It is best to avoid potted prawns, rich fish pâtés and fish roe as these are rich in saturated fat.

Shellfish contain higher levels of cholesterol but are low in saturated fat and may therefore be eaten in moderation – once or twice a week. Examples of shellfish are:

- cockles, mussels, whelks;

- shrimps, prawns, lobster;

- squid.

Fish oils can also be taken in the form of capsules. Oily fish have a particularly good effect in reducing triglycerides (see the section *Risks of high cholesterol levels* in Chapter 2), but some capsule preparations are high in calories, so be careful to check the label. Because of this, they have been known to upset people with diabetes and reduce the success of watching your weight. It is best to get your fish oil the natural way by regularly eating fish.

Omacor, a fish oil preparation, in addition to its benefit of reducing triglycerides, may be beneficial after a heart attack if added to statin therapy. The recommended dose is 1 g daily with food, and up to 4 capsules daily for raised triglycerides.

If I eat fish twice a week, will it allow me to eat what I like for the rest of the week?

No. A recent review of the scientific evidence about eating fish to protect against coronary artery disease concluded that 'merely adding fish to a nutritionally adverse diet will not grant a population immunity from epidemic coronary heart disease.' Translated this means that, if you are eating poorly, simply adding fish won't do any good. Fish should be part of a low saturated fat diet – part of a healthy eating plan.

I'm not keen on fish – can I have fish oil capsules instead?

Yes. Omacor and Maxepa lower triglycerides and Omacor has been shown to reduce the chances of further heart problems when taken after a heart attack and in addition to statins. Reduced hospital admissions for heart failure have also been recorded.

What is the difference between white fish and oily fish?

White fish includes cod, haddock, halibut, plaice and monkfish; oily fish includes herrings, kippers, mackerel, salmon, sardines, anchovies, trout and tuna. White fish is low in fat and this is good for the heart. Oily fish in addition contains a lot of omega-3 fatty acids as well as vitamins A and E, all of which may be good for the heart, so they have a greater potential benefit.

I quite like fish but it can be expensive. How much is it recommended that I eat each week?

The current recommendation is 300 g (12 oz) twice a week. The average intake in the UK is currently half this.

How do I know if the fish is fresh? I would hate to get food poisoning.

Fresh fish is usually refrigerated with ice before being sold but it can be frozen, then thawed, and sold as fresh. The law says it must be labelled as thawed because refreezing thawed fish is a source of bacteria. The safest way of buying or eating fish is to consume fresh fish within 24 hours of purchase or to cook frozen fish from frozen or immediately it has been thawed *for the first time.*

Fresh fish are usually stiff, the eyes are bright and not sunken, and the gills are red in colour. The skin should be shiny. Fillets should smell fresh (of the sea) and have firm moist flesh; white fillets look white and almost translucent in colour. If you are not sure, do not buy it and do not be convinced by the fishmonger as to its freshness unless you know him very well. Do not buy frozen fish which is not solid or has white patches or ice crystals on the skin. Frozen fish should not be thawed in water as it loses its texture, flavour and nutrients.

Independent fishmongers tend to know more about fish than supermarket fresh fish counter assistants.

Table 9.2 A guide to healthy eating*

Food types	Everyday foods
Cereals and breads	Flour and bread, pasta, breakfast cereals and porridge oats
Vegetables, fruit and pulses	Most kinds (fresh, dried, canned, frozen). Tofu and other soya products
Nuts	Nuts may be included in vegetarian diets to replace meats
Fish	Sardines, tuna, salmon, mackerel, trout, white fish (including haddock, cod, plaice) – steamed, grilled or baked, *not* fried
Meat	Chicken, turkey (both without skin), veal, lean ham
Eggs and dairy foods	Skimmed milk, cottage cheese, curd cheese, egg whites, low-fat yoghurt, low-fat fromage frais
Fats	All fats need to be limited
Preserves, spreads and sweets	Artificial sweeteners
Cakes, biscuits and desserts	Home-made cakes and biscuits made using low-fat recipes; jellies, sorbets, skimmed-milk puddings
Drinks	Tea, coffee, water, fruit juice, low-calorie soft drinks, clear soups
Other miscellaneous foods	Herbs, spices, mustard, vinegar, Worcester sauce, fat-free or low-fat salad dressings

* Information from *Trim the fat from your diet*, published by the British Heart Foundation

Eat in moderation	Eat with caution
Water biscuits; plain semi-sweet biscuits (e.g. rich tea, digestive) (once a week) cream crackers	Fancy bread and pastries, (e.g. croissants, brioches)
Chips and roast potatoes cooked in oil marked *High in polyunsaturates* or olive oil (once a fortnight); avocados, olives, lower-fat crisps (once a week)	Crisps, chips cooked in oil other than olive oil or oil marked *High in polyunsaturates*
Most nuts (use a few only)	Coconut
Shellfish (e.g. lobster, crab, prawns)	Any fish in batter, fish roe (e.g. taramasalata)
Not more than 3 times a week: lean cuts of beef, pork, lamb, bacon, lean mince; liver, kidney, meat paste	Visible fat on meat, sausages, pâté, duck, salami, meat pies and pasties, pork pies
Semi-skimmed milk; not more than 3 times a week: medium-fat cheese (such as Edam, Brie, Camembert, Parmesan); half-fat cheeses (e.g. half-fat Cheddar); 3–4 eggs a week	Full-cream milk, cream cheese, most blue cheeses (e.g. Stilton), full-fat yoghurt, condensed milk, cream, coffee creamers
Polyunsaturated margarines and oil (e.g. corn oil, sunflower oil, olive oil, low-fat spread)	Butter, dripping, lard, ghee, margarines not labelled *High in polyunsaturates*, blended vegetable oils
Jam, marmalade, honey, boiled sweets, fruit pastilles, sugar, peanut butter	Chocolates, toffees, fudge, mincemeat containing suet, chocolate spread
Occasional cakes, puddings and biscuits made with polyunsaturated margarine/oil (2–3 times a week), ice-cream	Ready-made cakes and biscuits, cream cakes, dairy cream, ice-cream, full-fat milk puddings
Packet soups, alcohol, low-fat drinking chocolate and malted drinks	Cream soups, full-fat milk drinks and shakes, cream-based drinks
Low-calorie salad cream and mayonnaise, French dressing made with polyunsaturated or olive oil	Salad cream, mayonnaise, creamy dressings

Isn't it possible to keep fresh fish in the fridge for a week?

Most fridges in our homes are set at about 3°C and fish spoils quickly at this temperature, so eat it within 24 hours. Stored on ice (0°C) fresh fish may last a week.

What types of food have low or high levels of fat and cholesterol in them?

Here are some of the main foods in the high fat groups.

Foods high in total fat

- Fried food
- Whole milk, cream, high-fat cheeses (such as Cheddar)
- Fatty meat and meat products, e.g. sausages and pâté

Foods high in saturated fat

- Fatty meat and meat products
- Foods cooked in lard, butter or hard margarines
- Cakes and pastries made with butter and hard margarines
- Palm and coconut oil
- Fatty poultry (duck, goose); poultry with the skin on

Foods high in total and LDL (bad) cholesterol

- Egg yolks (eat only three to four eggs a week at the most)
- Liver and other organ meats (kidney, brain, heart, sweetbreads)
- Shellfish (but these are lower in saturated fat than most meats and poultry so are fine to eat in moderation – see the question above on fish oils)

Foods high in polyunsaturated fat

- Some nuts and seeds (e.g. chestnuts, walnuts, not coconut)
- Oily fish
- Many soft margarines and vegetable oils (check the labels)

Foods high in monounsaturated fat

- Olive oil and olives
- Rapeseed oil
- Margarines and spreads made from olive oil

What sort of foods should I eat to cut down on my fat intake?

Basically, avoid full fat dairy produce, deep-fried foods, pastry, biscuits and puddings. See Table 9.2 for a comprehensive list of the healthiest foods to eat as regards fats, and those to eat in moderation, occasionally or best left alone. Don't panic – all the good things haven't been removed, it is just a modification as part of a new way of living.

For cutting down on dairy foods:

- Change whole milk dairy products to semi-skimmed or skimmed;
- Change butter or hard margarine to poly- or monounsaturated margarine;
- Change lard or hard vegetable fats to pure vegetable oils (such as corn oil or olive oil, high in polyunsaturates and monounsaturates respectively), but remember that all fats are high in calories;
- Change cream to low fat yoghurt or fromage frais;
- Change ice-cream to frozen yoghurt, sorbets or low fat frozen desserts;

- Change high fat cheeses (such as Cheddar, cream cheese) to lower fat cheeses (half fat Cheddar, Edam, Brie, Camembert, cottage cheese and lower fat soft cheese).

Eat no more than 170 g (6 oz) of cooked lean meat a day. If you do want to eat red meat:

- Eat the leaner cuts and always cut the fat off at the table;

- Avoid burgers, pork, meat pies, bacon and full fat sausages;

- Switch to chicken or turkey (but do not eat the skin);

- Switch to game meats instead of duck or goose which are fatty meats;

- Avoid processed meats (sausages, hot dogs, salami, pâté);

- Avoid high cholesterol organ meats (offal, e.g. liver, kidneys, sweetbreads).

Cut down on egg yolks (no more than three or four per week) or consider the use of egg substitutes or egg whites in cooking.

Eat fish that is low in saturated fat two or three times a week (you can include shellfish in moderation – see above). Try more oily fish than white fish.

Avoid purchased baked goods like cakes (substitute bread or muffins – but check the label) or meat pies.

Eat plenty of fresh fruit and vegetables, but avoid coconut, olives (not the oil) and avocados, which are high in calories and may cause weight gain).

Change from croissants to wholemeal bread.

Substitute chestnuts or walnuts for peanuts, but remember that all nuts contain a lot of calories.

According to the TV ads, some margarines seems to be a good way of lowering cholesterol – do they really work?

R esearch has shown that Benecol, which contains special plant extracts, lowers cholesterol by 10–14%. Similar results are reported with Flora Pro-activ. Although these products lower cholesterol, there is no evidence that they reduce heart risk in the same way that statin drugs do (see **Treatment** in the section **Risks of high cholesterol levels** in Chapter 2). They are helpful when you have a borderline raised cholesterol, because you may be able to avoid drugs; but, if you have heart disease already, these products should be used with drugs – you will then benefit from the drugs, but the doses might be lowered. I do recommend them as part of healthy living, but price may be a problem for some people, and you will get benefits from supermarket spreads that are high in either poly- or monounsaturated fats, if the costs worry you.

A liquid yoghurt drink a day maximises the benefit of Flora Pro-activ or Benecol.

My friend in America is taking nicotinic acid (niacin) for her cholesterol – is it available here?

N icotinic acid is available, but not often used because of its side effects, especially flushing. It can also affect the liver and make any stomach ulcers worse. It can react with alcohol and upset control in people with diabetes, so doctors have to monitor anyone on this drug very carefully. Occasionally, it can make angina pain worse.

A new formulation (Niaspan) has been launched. Nicotinic acid raises the good cholesterol (HDL) by up to 24%. Doctors will probably try it on those who have a low HDL in spite of being on statins, and therefore it is given in combination with these. Treatment will be introduced carefully and the dose gradually increased. Niaspan claims to cause less flushing than other types. Typical doses are 375, 500, 750 and 1000 mg, to a maximum of 2 g, taken daily at night. Flushing may be reduced by taking soluble aspirin 30 minutes beforehand and taking Niaspan with food.

Someone told me that nuts were good for reducing coronary disease – should I eat them regularly?

Nuts (though not coconut), eaten about four times a week, have been linked to a reduction in heart attacks. Walnuts and almonds lower cholesterol. Therefore, nuts as part of a healthy lifestyle may reduce the risk of heart disease. Eat them with cereals, as a snack, or with a salad. Beware of added salt and remember that they have a high calorie content. If you use nuts in cooking, remember some visitors may be allergic to them.

Are there better ways of cooking I could try?

Yes; instead of frying or roasting you could try grilling, barbecue-ing, braising, poaching, steaming, stir-frying or sautéing with minimal fat; baking, casseroling or microwaving also reduce the use of fats.

- Grill on a rack so that the fat drips away. Special fat-reducing portable grills are a healthy choice.

- If you have a roast, don't cook the meat in its own juice or make gravy from the juices. Cook the joint on a roasting rack and baste the meat with vegetable oil, lemon juice or a little olive oil.

- If you use a polyunsaturated margarine or oil for cooking, use as little as possible. Oil sprays are a way of avoiding excess in cooking.

Fibre

The doctor often recommends that I should eat more fibre. Is fibre important in my diet?

Fibre also means roughage; and yes, it is important. Most people associate roughage with bran but there are many foods which serve the same purpose (see Table 9.3). Starchy foods have the advantage that they are filling without providing a lot of calories. Fibre passes through the bowel without being absorbed into your body and lowers cholesterol by reducing fatty foods in your diet. This type of fibre, known as soluble fibre (see question below), is effective in lowering cholesterol, if enough is eaten. It binds with bile salts from

Table 9.3 Foods and fibre content

High fibre foods	Low fibre foods
Wholegrain cereals (branflakes, muesli, porridge, wheat biscuits)	Plain and frosted rice cereals, cornflakes, Special K
Breads (wholewheat, granary, rye, wholewheat pitta)	White bread and rolls
Brown rice, pearl barley, bulgur wheat	White rice
Pasta (wholewheat)	Pasta (white)
Wholewheat crispbread, crisprolls	White biscuits and crackers (water biscuits)
Popcorn, Twiglets, wholewheat breadsticks	Cheese Puffs, Hula Hoops, pretzels, Quavers
Wholewheat and oatmeal biscuits (especially with dried fruit)	Rich tea biscuits, shortbread, wafers
Wholemeal scones, fruited teabreads	Pastries, cakes

the liver, which are full of cholesterol, and prevents them from being absorbed. At the same time, by absorbing water like a sponge, it gives a full-up feeling.
Soluble fibre-rich foods include:

- pulse vegetables, e.g. peas, beans and lentils;

- fruit, e.g. bananas, apples, berries and citrus fruits; and

- oat cereals (not wheat).

The average person eats 15–20 g of fibre a day and this needs to be increased to over 25 g. As fibre is increased in the diet, it becomes important to drink plenty of fluids so that the swelling action can be achieved. Increase the fibre content gradually to give your digestive system a chance to adjust.

What is the difference between soluble and insoluble fibre? Should I eat both?

Insoluble fibre is important for digestion and taking it with fluid helps to prevent constipation and other bowel problems. Soluble fibre helps to lower cholesterol. Insoluble fibre is found in wholegrain and wholemeal foods (wholemeal bread, granary bread, brown rice, wholemeal or wholegrain flour and wholewheat breakfast cereals). A mixed diet of both types of fibre will keep you regular and lower your cholesterol.

When I am in the supermarket, I get confused as to which foods are best for fibre content. Can you tell me more about which contain more fibre?

To increase fibre is not difficult. Aim to eat two items from this list each mealtime:

- wholemeal bread or wholemeal chapattis or pitta bread;

- wholegrain cereal (bran, Weetabix, Shredded Wheat, porridge);

- baked potatoes (and eat the skins) instead of fried;

- wholegrain pasta and brown rice;

- fruit (particularly apples, pears, bananas): fruit is also low in calories and rich in vitamins and antioxidants (see the section *Risks of high cholesterol levels* in Chapter 2);

- dried fruit, e.g. raisins;

- vegetables (particularly root vegetables, e.g. carrots, turnips, parsnips; and green vegetables, e.g. sprouts, cabbage, broccoli): vegetables are also low in calories and rich in vitamins and antioxidants (see the section *Risks of high cholesterol levels* in Chapter 2);

- pulses: peas, beans, lentils, sweetcorn, baked beans, chickpeas;

- nuts: walnuts, chestnuts (but be careful, all nuts have a high calorie content).

Try to use wholemeal flour rather than white when you are baking, or a mixture. Table 9.3 gives a list of high versus low fibre foods.

I know that vegetables are good for me because they contain fibre and vitamins. I have heard that boiling vegetables loses the vitamins. How should I prepare fruit and vegetables to get the maximum benefits from them?

Many vitamins are lost in storage and on exposure to oxygen in the air. Buy (or pick) little and often and prepare just before you eat them. Leave the skin on where possible. Eat vegetables raw, or by steaming, stir-frying or microwaving. If you boil your vegetables, boil quickly in the minimum of water in a tightly covered pan and serve immediately. Use the cooking water for stock or gravy. Frozen vegetables are just as good as fresh and can be quick to prepare, convenient and economical.

Sugar

I have rather a sweet tooth. Is sugar really that bad for you?

Yes. Sugar is just calories without any good bits added (like vitamins, protein, fibre) and you get the calories that you need with the good bits by eating healthily. We really don't need sugar on its own as this can cause tooth decay. Sugary foods also tend to be high in calories, so eating too much can make you put on weight.

Chemical names for sugar are glucose, sucrose, fructose, dextrose and maltose. None is any better than another nor is brown or cane sugar any better than white.

I've read that poor dental health can cause coronary heart disease – is this true?

Poor dental health is not good for you whichever way you look at the problem. It causes bad breath and can lead to infections. There is a link between poor dental health and coronary heart disease but this may reflect other factors such as poor nutrition, cigarette smoking and generally poor conditions in a person's lifestyle. A recent publication has suggested that even allowing for these other factors, poor dental health can harm the heart. The message is clear – look after your teeth and gums!

Have you any tips for cutting down on sugar?

Cutting down on sugar is the easiest way to begin losing weight whereas cutting down on your fat intake is the most effective (see the section *Losing weight* below).

- Begin by cutting out sugar in tea and coffee. It may be tough at first but after four or five days you will wonder why you ever added sugar. Try to do without artificial sweeteners if you can, or use them only sparingly; some contain sodium (salt) which can upset your blood pressure control or treatment of heart failure.

- Drink low-calorie drinks, e.g. Diet Coke or caffeine-free diet coke, Diet 7-Up, diet tonic. Remember plain water is the most refreshing calorie-free drink there is.

- Choose tinned fruit in natural juice rather than syrup.

- Beware of sugar-coated breakfast cereals. A good breakfast could consist of low-fat, low-calorie yoghurt poured on unsweetened muesli, bran-type cereals with some fresh fruit, or porridge made with skimmed or semi-skimmed milk.

- Chocolate, cakes, biscuits and puddings can be replaced by fresh fruit, e.g. apples, bananas and pears, or low-fat yoghurts, fromage frais, low-fat mousses and frozen desserts.

Salt

I have raised blood pressure and my doctor tells me that I must cut down on my salt. Why is this?

Excess salt can raise the blood pressure (see Chapter 2). Salt (sodium chloride is the chemical name) in excess causes your body to retain water, upsetting the hormone balance, and the blood pressure goes up.

It is best to avoid extra salt at the table and any salty foods, e.g. crisps and salted nuts. Table 9.4 gives a guide to salty foods.

So how much salt do we actually need in our diet?

Your body needs 500 mg of sodium a day, the same as one-third of a teaspoon of salt. We eat on average one to three teaspoons of salt a day, equivalent to 6–18 g salt. In the UK, men eat just over 3 g sodium a day, equivalent to six to seven times more than they need.

Table 9.4 Levels of sodium in various foods

Foods	Typical portion size (g)	Sodium (mg)
Processed foods		
Bacon (grilled)	45	900
Baked beans	200	1060
Bread (2 slices)	75	390
Butter (salted, spread on large slice of bread)	7	61
Cereals		
All-Bran + milk	25 + 115	468
Cornflakes + milk	30 + 115	340
Cheddar cheese	30	183
Corned beef (2 slices)	60	570
Cream cracker + processed cheese	21 + 20	392
Ice-cream	75	54
Mars Bar	65	98
Pork pie (medium)	140	1104
Sausages (2 grilled)	90	900
Sausage roll		332
Scone	50	385
Spaghetti hoops	125	525
Tomato sauce (1 tbsp)	17	58
Tomato soup (canned)	240	1108
Unprocessed foods		
Apples (1 medium dessert, peeled)	120	2
Bananas (1 medium peeled)	100	1
Beef (roast topside, 3 slices)	90	43
Cabbage (boiled, white)	100	4
Carrots (boiled, old)	70	35
(tinned)	65	240
Chicken (meat only)	100	81
Cod in batter (fried)	85	85

Table 9.4 Levels of sodium in various foods (*continued*)

Foods	Typical portion size (g)	Sodium (mg)
Unprocessed foods (cont'd)		
Eggs (2, scrambled with milk/butter/salt)	140	1442
Potatoes (boiled, old)	150	5
(mashed with butter)	170	83
Drinks		
Beer (1 pint draught bitter)	568 ml	68
Bovril (heaped tsp)	5	240
Coffee (instant)	195	1
Horlicks + semi-skimmed milk	20 + 195	199
Marmite (heaped tsp)	5	225
Milk (2 tbsp)	30	15
Tea (1 cup)	195	Trace

I know that I eat too much salt and my blood pressure is on the high side. What foods should I try to limit?

When you read a food label, look at the sodium level not just the phrase 'low in salt' (see the questions on food labelling below). See the difference in processed foods which are high in sodium because salt is added during their manufacture (see Table 9.4). Salt gives us sodium – 1 g table salt contains 390 mg sodium. Now compare these with unprocessed foods which are low in sodium but high in potassium. Potassium is helpful in lowering blood pressure. Restriction of both sodium and potassium intake may be advised if you have kidney disease but healthy people usually get rid of any excess. However, if you eat a lot of sodium, this can lead to high blood pressure and fluid retention, which puts a strain on your heart.

Remember, there may be unexpected sources of salt – monosodium glutamate is often overlooked. Try herbs and spices rather than salt with your cooking. Watch out for salt in:

- snacks, especially salted nuts or crisps;
- frozen or canned fish (even tuna in brine);
- meat, especially ham or bacon, sausages, corned beef;
- canned foods and packet soups;
- commercial pies;
- some cheeses;
- salad dressings.

I have heard that bananas are very good for you. Why is this?

It is true to say that most people are not deficient in either sodium or potassium and a good healthy diet contains more potassium than most of us need. However, potassium-rich foods can help to lower blood pressure and may reduce the need for tablets in some people with high blood pressure. Many fruits like apples, pineapple, grapefruit and raw tomatoes contain potassium; dried raisins and bananas are particularly good sources. Leaf vegetables (spinach, broccoli, brussels sprouts, cabbage, celery and lettuce) are also good sources as are potatoes, parsnips, broad and baked beans. A high intake of potassium is not usually harmful because your kidneys get rid of any excess but, if you have kidney disease or are taking potassium-containing tablets, potassium levels can build up and cause irregular heartbeats. Check with your doctor if you are unsure.

How do I read food labels and what do the figures mean for me?

It is important to know about salt, fat and calories. Most of the salt that you eat is that added in food manufacturing, so simply watching the salt you add is not enough. Some food labels may specify the sodium content, but it would be impracticable (and difficult) for you to have to add up the sodium content of all manufactured foods that you buy. As a general guide, cut down on salt added in cooking, avoid it at the table and avoid the very salty foods listed above.

Try to keep your daily cholesterol below 300 mg and sodium below 3000 mg (3 g). This is a higher sodium intake than we need but the body copes with this and it is a more practical approach to food. Sodium in grams × 2.5 equals salt in grams; so, 3 g of sodium = 7.5 g of salt and 2.4 g of sodium = 6 g salt. We need 500 mg of sodium a day (500 mg = 0.5 g) and that equals 1.25 g salt or one-third of a teaspoon.

As a reminder, your fat intake varies with calorie advice but for a typical female, who needs 2000 kcal a day, this will be about 70 g of fat, and for a male needing 2500 kcal a day, 95 g of fat. Of these figures, saturated fat should be no more than a third. Table 9.5 is adapted from the American Heart Association Guidelines.
Here are some guidelines for reading labels.

- Compare figures per 100 g and per serving if you eat the whole pack. You can usually compare product to product per 100 g.

- For each 100 g portion, a simple guide to content is shown in Table 9.6.

- Energy is measured in calories (kilocalories shortened to kcal) and joules (kilojoules shortened to kJ): 1 kcal equals 4.2 kJ.

Table 9.5 Guidelines for food intake
for average-sized men and women per day

Intake	Men	Women
Energy	2500 kcal	2000 kcal
Total fat*	95 g	70 g
Saturated fat[†]	30 g	20 g
Fibre	20 g	16 g
Salt[‡]	6.0 g	5.5 g

* Total fat is 35% of energy.
[†] Total saturated fat is 11% of energy.
[‡] 6.0g salt equals 2 level teaspoons and 2.4g sodium.

If you take in more calories than you burn up, you will gain weight. See above for your daily needs.

- Proteins are important for your body's building bricks. We all have more than we need except vegetarians, who need to pay more attention to increasing the protein content of their diet to adequate levels.

- Sugar content should be no more than 70 g daily for men and 50 g for women.

An example of a good food label, giving us all the essential information, is given in Table 9.7. Look at the fat, fibre, sugar and sodium content and compare with Table 9.6.

Garlic

I have read that garlic is very good for high blood pressure. Is this true?

There is unfortunately no evidence that garlic reduces cholesterol but it may slightly reduce blood pressure – more research is needed. The best advice is to make garlic part of your diet, providing, of course, that you like it and it doesn't limit your social life!

Drinks

I drink quite a few cups of coffee a day. Is coffee bad for the heart?

High caffeine levels can cause palpitations (see Chapter 6). Boiled coffee (percolators) can raise cholesterol but instant, filter or expresso do not. There is no real evidence of any harmful effect of coffee on the coronary arteries. So you can drink and enjoy coffee without worrying about it causing a heart attack. Try to avoid percolated coffee because of the cholesterol effect and cut down on all coffee if you have palpitations.

Table 9.6 Guide to food-type content in 100 g-portions

Food type	A lot (g)	A little (g)
Sugar	10	2
Fat	20	3
Saturated fats	5	1
Fibre	3	0.5
Sodium	0.5	0.1

I like to have a drink now and again. How does alcohol affect my heart?

Alcohol in moderation helps the heart, but in excess it can cause strokes, high blood pressure and cirrhosis of the liver. Alcohol therefore can be consumed without undue worry but it needs to be controlled. Alcohol is, unfortunately, high in calories, so it is not helpful if you are trying to lose weight. Binge drinking is very bad for blood pressure – the following day your blood pressure may be very high and this is when strokes occur.

We measure alcohol in terms of units and it is recommended that men have no more than 28 and women 21 units in a week. Ideally men should not drink more than 4 units a day and women 3 units a day. The British Heart Foundation recommends a weekly limit of 21 units for men and 14 for women. When pouring drinks at home no one ever pours a single shot of spirits unless they use an actual measure – it is always a double or even a treble!

To calculate a unit, multiply the strength of the drink by its volume and divide by 1000. So 250 cc of wine, as often served in wine bars, of 10% strength, is 2.5 units ($250 \times 10 \div 1000$).

One unit of alcohol is equal to:

- one 100 cc glass of wine (red or white): a typical 125 ml measure represents 1.6 units per glass (a bottle of wine at 12.5% volume contains six 125 ml glasses);

- a single measure of sherry;
- half a pint of normal strength beer;
- quarter of a pint of strong beer;
- a single measure of a spirit.

Table 9.7 An example of a good food label for a breakfast cereal

Ingredients: Wheat, malt extract, sugar, salt, niacin, iron, thiamin (B1), riboflavin (B2), folic acid

Nutrition information

	Typical values per 100 g (3.5 oz)	*Typical values per 37.5 g serving with 150 ml semi-skimmed milk*
Energy	339 kcal	191 kcal
	1439 kJ	811 kJ
Protein	11.5 g	9.1 g
Carbohydrates	67.3 g	31.7 g
of which Sugars	4.7 g	9.2 g
Starch	62.6 g	22.5 g
Fat 2.7 g	3.4 g	
of which Saturates	0.7 g	1.8 g
Mono-unsaturates	0.3 g	0.9 g
Polyunsaturates	1.7 g	0.6 g
Fibre	10.9 g	3.9 g
Sodium	0.3 g	0.2 g
Thiamin (B1)	1.2 mg (85% RDA)	0.5 mg (35% RDA)
Riboflavin (B2)	1.4 mg (85% RDA)	0.8 mg (47% RDA)
Niacin	15.3 mg (85% RDA)	5.7 mg 31% RDA)
Folic acid	170 µg (85% RDA)	70.0 µg (35% RDA)
Iron 11.9 mg (85% RDA)	4.4 mg (31% RDA)	

RDA means Recommended Daily Allowance
Per 37.5 g serving with 150 ml semi-skimmed milk = 191 calories and 3.4 g fat

Any form of alcohol benefits the heart (not just red wine) but it must be at a regular acceptable intake – you can't save all your units up for Saturday night! See also the question below on calories in alcohol. Some alcohol now has the units on the can or bottle – this is very helpful and more labels should carry this information.

Always make sure alcohol does not interfere with any medication you might be taking. For example, it increases the effect of warfarin and it interacts with sleeping tablets (increasing their effects) and some painkillers (e.g. co-codamol) and some antibiotics (such as metronidazole). Alcohol can also increase the drowsiness some people experience with antihistamines (such as Piriton).

I have heard a lot about the benefits of wine. Is wine better than beer or spirits?

Unfortunately, this has become confusing with reports contradicting each other. All alcohol is beneficial in moderation. Wine has some advantages over beer. However, alcohol is *not* a medicine and should only be taken if enjoyed.

Snacks

Besides fruit can you suggest some healthy snacks?

Here are some ideas to try.

For nibbles

- raw vegetables (cucumber, celery, mangetout, baby corn, broccoli or cherry tomatoes)
- dried fruits (apricots, banana, raisins, sultanas)
- yoghurt (low-fat types)
- popcorn (no added salt or sugar)

For more substantial snacks

- fresh vegetable soups (not cream)

- beans on toast

- baked potatoes (fill with cottage cheese, baked beans or salad)

- wholemeal or soft grain white bread sandwiches with healthy fillings, e.g. tuna and sweetcorn, turkey and salad, a little Brie cheese and fruit

Drink water, slimline tonic or tea with lemon or lime.

All these suggestions are not only good for a healthy diet, but also a good way towards losing weight (see section below).

LOSING WEIGHT

It is easy to start cutting down on calories but keeping to your resolutions is tough. Most people with high blood pressure tend to be overweight. **Losing weight should be a gradual process as part of a lifestyle change – avoid dramatic slimming fads.**

I know I have to lose some weight. Have you any general tips?

Most people know what is fattening and what isn't so you can avoid obvious foods (see Table 9.2) but here are a few tips.

- Losing weight is much easier if at the same time you increase your physical exercise. Taking exercise benefits the heart in general (see Chapter 10). To lose weight you need to take a brisk walk, or an equivalent form of exercise, for 60–90 minutes daily.

- Avoid snacking. If you nibble a lot, drink plenty of water, and use fruit or starchy foods (such as a roll with low fat spread) as your filler rather than peanuts or crisps. See the list above for healthy snacks.

- Plan your meals and plan how to avoid temptation. If you are visiting friends for a meal let them know what you are trying to achieve and why. Good friends will be pleased that you confided in them – they will probably be constructive and helpful. If you go to a restaurant, look for those which have courses that fit in with your healthy eating plan.

- If you develop a craving (a choc attack!), reach for that apple and go for a walk. Remind yourself what you are doing and why.

- If you slip, don't give up, regroup and get back on course.

- Avoid too much alcohol – instead of a gin and tonic have a slimline tonic. Have one glass of wine, not two. (See the question below on alcohol.)

- Eat slowly and take your time over the meal.

- Have a salad (with a low-calorie dressing) with the meal.

- Always eat breakfast. Porridge is a good low-calorie filler. Use semi-skimmed milk. Cereals vary a lot as regards calorie content – read the label carefully rather than the marketing message.

- Don't miss meals or have one big meal a day.

- Don't shop when you are hungry and always take a shopping list with you rather than go for impulse buying.

- Use a smaller plate when serving.

- Stick a photograph of *how you want to be* on the fridge. It will help you to avoid temptation as you visualise the new slimmer you!

- Slim with a friend or join a reputable slimming club – group support can be very motivating.

- Eat healthy foods (as discussed in the section *Food types and eating healthily* above).

- Always cut the fat off food and do not cook in fat. Avoid fried foods. (See the advice above on the best ways to cook food.)

- If you do use fat for cooking, use a healthier oil (such as olive oil) which is high in unsaturated fats (see Chapter 2). Shallow-fry in the minimum of oil to get the maximum benefit. Use a non-stick frying pan and do not overheat. If you deep fry, use a 'good' oil and replace the oil after five uses.

- Keep away from cakes, milk chocolate, biscuits and any pastries or pies (dark chocolate in moderation may be beneficial).

- Choose plainer biscuits, e.g. rich tea or marie types.

- Have a fresh fruit salad, fruit tinned in natural juices, fromage frais, low-fat mousse or frozen yoghurt for dessert.

How quickly should I lose weight?

Aim for no more than 1 kg (2 lb) a week – a gradual change is more likely to be sustained and it is healthier.

My friend has taken so-called diet tablets. Do these work?

Eating healthily and weight loss are about making lifestyle changes, so drugs should be avoided if at all possible. Some drugs are addictive and others may damage the heart valves. Many that are sold for high prices are capsules of nonsense. Xenical (orlistat), however, has research behind it. It may help obese people as part of a lifestyle change. It goes with a properly controlled low-fat diet and works by inhibiting the absorption of 30% of the fat eaten. Side effects include bowel disturbances. Xenical is part of a carefully controlled diet, supervised by a dietitian, and is a course of tablets, not a long-term treatment. It is not a magic slimming bullet, but it does have an important role for a small number of obese people.

Rimonabant acts on the brain to reduce the craving for food and has been an effective weight-reducing drug when used in combination with taking dietary advice. It can lead to depression, causing its marketing to be halted. Not everyone benefits from drug therapy but drugs can help a significant number of people.

I have been on a slimming diet and managed to lose some weight. How can I keep the weight off now?

First of all remember why you lost it – you have lowered your blood pressure and reduced the strain on your heart. So praise yourself. You will feel better and that alone will give you the incentive you need to keep slim and fit.

Here are some more tips.

- Maintain regular exercise, walking briskly, cycling, swimming (see Chapter 10).

- Keep eating sensibly: plan your meals and follow the plan carefully.

- Eat more starchy foods (such as an extra slice or two of bread a day) to prevent you losing more weight if you have reached your target. Do not be tempted to turn to biscuits and cakes again!

- At parties or business lunches, if there is a buffet, choose carefully and don't overeat just because its free and the size of the spread is tempting (see question below on eating out).

- If hunger strikes, drink a glass of water and eat fruit – don't open the fridge door.

If you start gaining weight, look carefully at what you are eating and how much you exercise – what have you changed? If you lose weight below your target, gradually increase your calorie intake first of all by 200 kcal a day (an apple is 60 kcal, a slice of bread 80 kcal: there are many 'calorie counting' booklets on the market, listing various foods both raw and packaged); after a week, check it again and keep exercising.

I have seen two different charts for an ideal weight. What should my target weight be?

Your ideal weight must take into account your height (see Figure 9.1). Doctors work to your Body Mass Index or BMI. This is your weight in kilograms divided by the square of your height in metres:

$$\text{BMI} = \frac{\text{weight in kg}}{(\text{height in metres})^2} = \frac{\text{kg}}{\text{m}^2}$$

A normal BMI is 20–25. It works well for people over 1.6 m (5 ft 3 in) up to 1.87 m (6 ft 2 in) but not so well for short or tall people. Ask your doctor or practice nurse to help you work out your BMI and set your own target BMI. Now check it against your bathroom scales which are not as accurate but which will still show any changes. You can work out what you weigh in kilograms which is equally a guide to your BMI. For example, say that your BMI is 27 and that you want to get to 25, work out your kg at each BMI point and then, using your bathroom scales, all you need to do is set your kg target, as you know what BMI it represents. If you are not sure what to do or how to do it, ask the practice nurse to help you. Here is an example to help you:

A 1.87 m (6 ft 2 in) man weighs 95 kg. His calculated BMI is:

$$\frac{95}{1.87 \times 1.87} = 27.2$$

He would like to be healthier with a BMI of 24–25 so the calculation is:

$$24 = \frac{? \text{ kg}}{1.87 \times 1.87} \quad \text{i.e. 84 kg}$$

He now knows what to aim for on his scales.

Check your weight once a week only and aim to lose 1 kg (2.2 lb) in the first week and then 0.5 kg a week thereafter. If you use bathroom scales, do not put them on a carpet, and check them against a known weight (such as bags of flour) from time to time. Compare them with your doctor's scales or a large one in a chemist's shop.

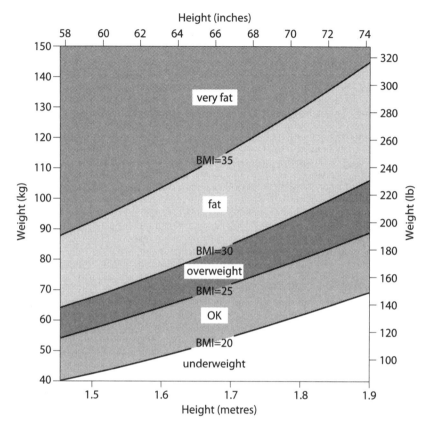

Use the chart or do this calculation to find out your BMI: divide your weight in kilograms by the square of your height in metres.

Your BMI score:
below 20: underweight
20–25: ideal
25–30: overweight
30+: seriously overweight – you need to see your doctor

Figure 9.1 What you should weigh. Take a straight line up from your height (without shoes) and across your weight (without clothes), and put a mark where the lines meet. How did you do?

I find the whole business of BMI confusing – can it be made simpler?

Of course. Simply follow the height and weight chart. Another simple formula is:

- Height in cm minus 110 = optimal weight in kg for men
- Height in cm minus 100 = optimal weight in kg for women.

So, if you are male measuring 5 ft 10 in, convert your height to centimetres (177.8 cm), take away 110 and you reach 67.8 kg. This is your ideal weight.

I have heard the nurse talk about a waist/hip ratio. What is this? Does it apply to my husband as well as me?

If your tummy is fat, the risk of heart problems increases and you can calculate the risk by comparing the waist measurement with that at the hip. You divide your waist measurement by your hip measurement. So, if your waist measures 26 in and hip 34 in, then you would have a ratio of 0.76 (26 divided by 34); you would not be at risk because the safe ratio for women should be no more than 0.8; this means that your waist should not be more than 80% of your hip measurement. Put another way, being apple-shaped is bad but pear-shaped is positively good!

The ratio for your husband, say with a 40 in waist and a 34 in hip, is calculated by dividing 40 by 34 which equals 1.18. He would be at risk because the safe ratio for men should be no more than 1.0. So his waist should not be greater than his hip measurement or the ratio would be over 1.0. Having a belly that's bigger than your hips increases your risks of getting coronary artery disease.

Waist circumference is used more as a sign of obesity and predisposition to diabetes. It is measured breathing out, 2 cm (1 in) above the umbilicus (navel). For men, if your waist is 94–102 cm (37–40 in) you are overweight; over 102 cm (40 in) and you are fat (politely known as obese). In women, if the waist is 80–88 cm

(32–35 in) you are overweight, and over 88 cm (35 in) you are fat. Doctors tend to focus more on abdominal obesity which increases the risk of heart disease.

I've tried all sorts of slimming diets and nothing seems to work – what can I do now?

Trying a slimming diet is not the right way of tackling weight reduction – it is a lifestyle change that is needed. If you cannot do it on your own, don't give up. Join one of the groups such as WeightWatchers and attend regularly. Remember why you need to lose weight: your blood pressure will benefit and you will reduce your chances of a stroke or heart attack.

Is it safe for heart patients to try the Atkins diet?

The Atkins diet is high fat, high protein and low carbohydrate. The theory is that when we eat carbohydrates and sugar the body responds by making insulin to burn them off. Too much intake equals too much insulin and then too much fat is stored and therefore we gain weight. In the short term it works for many people but there is a tendency towards constipation and bad breath. Heart patients with high cholesterol levels are usually protected by statins but control can be lost. My view is that if there is significant weight loss, this is good in the short term – say 2–3 months – but for long-term protection a switch should be made to the Mediterranean Diet, which is proven to cut the risks of a heart attack and is the programme described in this chapter.

We have a local WeightWatchers group in our area. Are slimming groups any good?

Any group like this can be helpful because of the supportive role and the sensible advice they offer. They reinforce the following basic rules.

- Eat less fat and sugar.
- Avoid nibbles.
- Do not miss meals.
- Eat more fruit and vegetables.
- Fill up on low-fat high fibre foods.
- Take regular dynamic exercise, e.g. walking, cycling, swimming – any strong movement exercise.

You have mentioned before that Asians have a higher incidence of coronary disease and diabetes – what dietary changes can they make?

It is true that Asians in particular are vulnerable to coronary disease and diabetes, and have a tendency to abdominal obesity. Try the following tips.

- Fried foods should be avoided.
- Eat low-fat yoghurt, semi-skimmed or skimmed milk and reduced fat cheeses instead of full-fat versions.
- Try casseroling, boiling, grilling, steaming, poaching or microwave cooking instead of adding fat or oil. Some vegetables, such as fenugreek (methi), aubergines and karelas, soak up more oil in during cooking.
- Try to make minced meat dishes and dhals without fat and avoid using oil in the cooking.
- Remove visible fat from meats.
- Do not spread fat on chapattis and do not add oil or ghee to the chapatti dough.
- Reduce deep fried snacks, e.g. chevdon, sev, samosas, puris, pakoras and chips.

- Switch from creamy salad dressing to low-fat yoghurt based dressing.

There is an excellent information sheet on this website: www.heartuk.org.uk (number 03).

We have a full social life and I am often out during the week at business lunches. How can I avoid fatty foods when I am out?

If you are going to family or friends, tell your host that you have been told to lose weight and what you need to do about it. They will understand and because they will now know that you don't eat fatty foods or sweet desserts, any embarrassment will be avoided.
The following tips apply to eating in restaurants.

- Avoid the cocktails (tomato juice and mineral water are just as fashionable these days).

- Avoid fried appetisers or cream soups – select minestrone or gazpacho soups.

- Choose a fresh fruit starter such as melon.

- Look for the grilled fish or poultry and ask for any sauces to be left off.

- Grilled Dover sole and a salad are a good standby.

- Remove the skin from poultry and don't eat fatty meat.

- Take a salad with vinegar and oil instead of mayonnaise.

- At a salad bar, avoid cream dressings, cheese, olives, bacon bits and croûtons.

- Have fresh vegetables such as spinach or carrots. Ask for sauces or butter to be left off vegetables or put 'on the side'.

- Order baked or boiled new potatoes in their skins.

- At Oriental restaurants, have a stir-fry of chicken or fish and vegetables. Steamed rice is better than fried. Resist sweet 'n sour dishes and banana or apple fritters.

- In Italian restaurants, avoid creamy sauces.

- In Indian restaurants, have plain tandoori or tikka with a salad and steamed or boiled rice, rather than those dishes which come in thick sauces. Indian cooking involves a lot of fat and sometimes coconut so, in general, menu options should be very carefully selected. Ask if you are not sure how certain dishes are cooked.

- Dessert can be fresh fruit or sorbet – try to avoid cream.

- Enjoy a glass of wine and perhaps finish with black coffee (decaffeinated if you are prone to palpitations – see Chapter 6).

Some restaurants now have items marked as being low in fat. Airlines also often offer this when meal options are presented.

If you are the host, you can choose the restaurant. If you are a regular at a particular restaurant, tell the owner about your preferences so that you will be able to eat without drawing attention to any question mark over your health.

There are times when I really fancy a steak. Should I never eat this?

An occasional treat is fine. Make sure it is a grilled fillet with the fat removed. If you are not sure what to eat, always go for the healthy option but, if after a while you feel you 'could murder a steak', enjoy one, but don't overdo it. Remember, a 170–225 g (6–8 oz) fillet steak is the best weight to go for.

What should my intake of fats be?

Your saturated fat intake should represent no more than 10% of your total calories; polyunsaturated fats should make up 10% and monounsaturated fats 10–15%. As 1 g of fat equals 9 kcal:

- if your daily calorie intake is 1500 kcal, you need only 50 g of fat at most;

- if it is 2000 kcal you need 65–70 g of fat, and

- if it is 2500 kcal, you need 85–90 g of fat.

Can you give some simple guidelines regarding calories?
How many should I need on a daily basis?

To calculate the number of calories to maintain your weight now, multiply the number of pounds you weigh by 13 kcal if you don't take much exercise, and by 15 if you do. The equivalent figures if you calculate in kilograms are 29 and 33 respectively.

To lose 1 lb you need to burn up 3500 kcal (7700 kcal for 1 kg) and this means reducing your daily intake by 500 kcal to lose 1 lb in one week (550 kcal for 0.5 kg). You can cut down 500 kcal by, for example, cutting out a can of coke, a chocolate bar or 4 teaspoons of sugar.

Weigh yourself once a week and adjust your intake accordingly. Always combine weight loss with a healthy increase in physical activity. For example, if you walk briskly at 4 miles per hour for 2 miles, you will use up 300 kcal.

If you fall below your target weight, increase your calorie intake by 200 kcal a day (around a couple of slices of bread and a thin slice of lean ham) but keep up the exercise programme.

I know I should eat more vegetables and fruit in my diet to lose
weight. Which ones have the least calories?

Nearly all vegetables and fruits in general are low in calories and high in nutrients and vitamins. However, dried fruits are high in calories. Vegetables are encouraged because they are very nutritious and low in calories, so you can really go to town with them! Some, especially beans and legumes, are packed with protein and great for using instead of meat dishes (as in lentil lasagne) or to pad out meat-based meals (as in chilli con carne). You do not really need to count the calories but, as a guide, an average portion of the following vegetables is equal to about 20 kcal:

Asparagus	Mushrooms
Aubergine	Onions
Green beans	Parsnips
Broccoli	Peas
Brussels sprouts	Peppers
Cabbage	Radishes
Carrots	Spinach
Cauliflower	Tomatoes
Celery	Turnips
Cucumber/courgette	Vegetable juices
Lettuce	

The following fruits are each equal to 60 kcal:

1 apple	1 nectarine
4 apricots	1 orange
1 banana	1 peach
12 cherries	3 dates
2 plums	2 figs
3 prunes	½ grapefruit
2 tangerines	15 grapes
2 tablespoons of raisins	½ mango
1 portion blackberries/melon/ pineapple/strawberries/raspberries	

If you buy tinned fruit, make sure that they are in natural juices, not syrup.

What exactly is a 'portion'?

A portion is one large fruit (such as an apple, orange or banana); two small fruits (such as plums or satsumas); 1 cup of raspberries, strawberries or grapes; 1 glass (150 ml) of fruit juice; 1 tbsp of dried fruit; 2 tbsp of raw, cooked or frozen vegetables or 1 dessert bowl of salad.

*I know there is a good deal of fibre in breads and cereals.
What about their calorie value?*

The following are equal to 80 kcal:

- 1 slice of bread;

- 1 portion of bran cereal (such as All-Bran, one Shredded Wheat) without milk;

- 1 portion of pasta or rice.

Remember that high fibre starchy foods are valuable parts of a healthy lifestyle as we have already discussed.

How many calories are there in alcohol?

A glass of wine is 100 kcal, a pint of beer 400 and a single measure of spirit 100, whereas slimline tonic is at most 1 calorie and water contains nil. Unsweetened fresh fruit juice and sparkling water are very good alternatives to alcohol when you are trying to watch your weight.

I want to be healthy and not overweight – can you summarise for me the most important ways of achieving this?

It is important to think of any change as a healthy change to your lifestyle. Losing weight must be a part of a change to healthy food and a regular exercise programme. It is really a healthy way of living rather than just losing weight. To achieve this, follow these basic rules.

- Eat lots of fruit and vegetables every day.

- Eat high fibre foods which are filling, healthy and low in fat.

- Try to avoid fatty foods, e.g. bacon, sausages and pies.

- When you have poultry, do not eat the skin.

- Avoid cakes and crisps, which contain a lot of fat.

- Use low-fat yoghurt or fromage frais instead of cream.

- When you cook, steam, grill, bake or microwave food instead of frying.

- When you have canned fish, drain off the oil (your cat would like it) or use those that come in brine.

- When you have pasta, use tomato-based vegetable sauce rather than creamy sauces.

- When you use fats, even polyunsaturated or olive oil, use it sparingly.

- Try not to nibble nuts.

- Eat slowly.

- Use a smaller plate.

- Cut down on alcohol; drink plenty of water.

- Don't replace meals by snacks – always eat breakfast.

- Don't shop when you are hungry.

- Don't be depressed if you slip up – regroup and start again the next day.

- Try to take dynamic exercise three times a week for at least 30 minutes.

If I miss a meal because I am travelling or I am on business, what can you suggest as an alternative?

Cereal bars, fig rolls, nuts, oat biscuits and rice cakes provide low-fat energy. Fruit is always a good standby – an apple a day may well keep the doctor away after all!

10 | Exercise

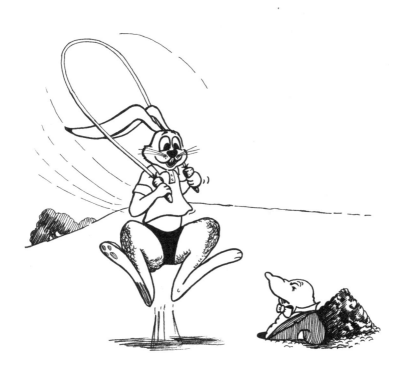

WHY BOTHER?

Most people get little vigorous exercise either at work or during their leisure time. We travel by car, bus or train, and at the end of the day we flop down in front of the TV. There is now a lot of evidence that regular exercise of low or moderate intensity, done on a regular basis (daily if possible, four to five times a week otherwise), can reduce the risk of getting heart disease. Activities that benefit the heart include walking, climbing stairs, gardening, housework such as making the beds or vacuuming the stairs (and not just wafting a feather duster), dancing or using home or gym exercise equipment. Increasing your exercise to be more vigorous helps further improve your heart and lungs – brisk walking, cycling, swimming, skipping or running (jogging) are examples of easy exercise that can become part of your everyday lifestyle.

Throughout this book the importance of exercise for the heart has been stressed. It really does help to be fit. If you find it a struggle to exercise on your own, get the whole family to join in and be supportive. Otherwise, try the following ideas.

- Join a sports or leisure club.

- Do any exercise that you enjoy.

- Try a new sport such as golf.

- Clean your car yourself, not in a car wash.

- Get working in the garden if you have one – 30 minutes in the fresh air digging or weeding is excellent exercise.

- Go swimming with a friend or relative.

- Get the bicycle out of storage; have it serviced if necessary, and buy the right safety kit; try it out on a quiet road at first if you don't feel confident.

- If you have an exercise bicycle, stop hanging clothes on it and start using it.

- Don't give up – every little helps.

- Keep working at it.

- Always be positive.

Remember that exercise should be enjoyed, not endured. You should be able to find some form of exercise that you really enjoy.

Why will exercise do me good?

There are many reasons why exercise is so good for everyone:

- It will help you lose and maintain your optimal weight.
- It increases your 'good' cholesterol (HDL).
- It helps smokers stop smoking.
- It lowers blood pressure and thus helps prevent heart disease.

Physically fit people are usually psychologically fit also. Fit people feel better, live longer and have less heart disease and diabetes. They also sleep better and handle stress better.

What types of exercise are good for the heart? I have been doing weight lifting for years – is it of any help to my heart?

Activities that involve movement (walking, cycling, swimming) are known as dynamic or aerobic exercise and these are the ones that benefit the heart. Aerobic means that the body uses oxygen to deliver the energy that you need for the activity that you are performing. Aerobic exercise for at least 30 minutes four or five times a week will strengthen your heart and help to reduce your chance of developing coronary artery disease.

Weight lifting is a form of static exercise, also known as isometric or akinetic exercise. This does not help the heart and can put on unnatural strain on it by raising your blood pressure. Other examples of static exercise are pushing a car that won't start, lifting heavy bags without help, moving furniture on your own – you know that with a big effort you can do it, but if you wait for help there will less strain on your heart.

Building up your muscles without dynamic exercise may make the outside of your chest look good but it will not help the heart inside. Those ill-advised people who take steroids can actually damage their heart because steroids sometimes weaken the heart muscle so that it becomes flabby. Anabolic steroids can cause the blood to clot more easily and a heart attack becomes more likely.

I've read about exercise and there is often a mention of METs – what are they?

A MET is short for 'metabolic equivalent'. This is a measure of the work the body does when exercising – the more you work at exercise, the more METs you use. Sitting watching the TV equals 1 MET, walking will use up to 5 METs depending on how brisk it is, and running will use even more (see Table 10.1). When we exercise we achieve our personal limit depending on how fit we are, and this is known as our 'functional capacity'. As our fitness improves, so does our functional capacity.

If I'm fit why should I quit smoking as well?

No risk factor works on its own. Getting fit goes along with losing weight, not smoking, avoiding fatty foods and moderating alcohol. If you smoke you are three times more likely to get coronary artery disease. Smoking is a bigger cause of heart disease than lack of exercise. So if you are super fit but smoke 10–20 cigarettes a day, the smoking will win the argument and you will lose out – being fit does not allow you to smoke.

I am now 51 and made a resolution on my 50th birthday to take exercise regularly. I found that my good intentions fell away after 3 months when I was ill for a week with flu. What do you suggest might help now?

First of all it is important not to exercise when you are ill, so you did the right thing when you had flu. Start again with a practice walk for about a mile, going slowly, then try and reduce the time that this length takes. Keep a record. If you walk on a footpath by a roadway, you can measure the distance using a car;

Table 10.1 Activities and their metabolic equivalents

Activity	METs
Aerobics	
low impact	5
high impact	7
Badminton	4.5
Bowling	4
Cycling	
< 10 mph	4
10–12 mph	6
> 12 mph	10
DIY (e.g. wallpapering)	4–5
Football	8
Gardening (e.g. digging)	3–5
Golf	4–5
Horse riding (trotting)	5–7
Housework (average)	2.5
scrubbing floors	5.5
Playing the piano	2.5
Office job	1.5
Sex ('normal')	2–3
Sex ('vigorous')	3–6
Skiing	
downhill racing	8
leisure	6
Squash	12
Swimming	
fast	10
moderate	8
light	6
butterfly	11
Table tennis	4
Tennis	8
Walking (1 mile in 20 min)	3

if you walk in the countryside, select a path where the distance is shown.

If you walk for 1 mile at 2 mph, you will take 30 minutes and use up 2.5 METs, which isn't much effort but it is an important beginning. At 3 mph it will take you 20 minutes and use 3.5 METs; at 4 mph it will take 15 minutes and use 4.5 METs. When you are walking fast and just out of breath, fitness will be achieved for the over-40s at about 5 METs for men and women – this is equivalent to walking 2 miles in 30 minutes.

I'm over 60 and have never really taken exercise properly, though I live an outdoor life. Am I too old to exercise now?

Age should not be a limitation to anybody starting to take exercise although it is better to have exercised throughout your life. Exercise will keep you feeling and looking younger longer. If you haven't exercised before or are starting again after a long gap, just remember to build up gradually. Always check with your doctor first, if you are at all uncertain as to whether a particular form of exercise is suitable for you.

I am going to start an exercise routine. How will I be able to work out how many calories I use up?

This depends on the type of exercise you take and for how long.

- If you walk at 3 miles an hour (about normal walking speed), you will burn up 320 kcal per hour.

- If you walk at 4.5 mph (pretty fast, almost a jog), this goes up to 440 kcal per hour.

- If you cycle at 6 mph, you will burn 240 kcal per hour.

- If you swim 25 yards (a length of most swimming pools) in a minute, you will burn 275 kcal per hour.

The fatter you are, the more you burn, and you burn more if you exercise for longer rather than faster; for example cycling at 12 mph burns 410 kcal per hour not 480.

HOW MUCH?

I have a busy life and am not sure that I can set aside half an hour every day for exercising. Is my effort wasted if I do not take exercise every day?

You must begin slowly – you cannot become an athlete overnight – and increase gradually. The aim is to perform any aerobic exercise for 30–40 minutes four to five times a week. Even relatively modest exercise is good, e.g. gardening, housework and dancing, but it is better if you can develop a walking programme to include both distance and speed as well as enjoyment (see below for a good programme to follow).

Try to exercise at least every other day and more at the weekend (a walk in the country at the weekend will be fun and less polluted than a city walk). Try to make it a regular commitment, such as every lunch hour, especially if your workplace offers showers. Afterwards, have a glass of water. Ask a friend or partner to join in. Keep a record to judge your progress. Dancing can be quite vigorous (such as country dancing), so it is a particularly good form of exercise because you can build up from gentler beginnings. It is also exercise with a good social side to it.

I am put off exercising because, in my exercise class, everyone else seems much fitter than me. Why is this?

Life is like that! At first everyone seems fitter: they may have been working at it longer. They were probably unfit once and so they will be supportive. You are the most important person and you should focus purely on your own programme. Don't worry about what everybody else is doing. It is not a competition. Don't be embarrassed, get stuck in.

SAFETY

You mention talking to my doctor before I start exercising. Do I really need a medical check first?

If you have no medical problems, the answer is no – get out and start straight away. If you've already had heart trouble or don't know about your blood pressure, get this checked by your doctor and ask for a cholesterol check while you are there. If you are 'at risk' (over 60 years, a smoker, have diabetes or on medication for your heart), it's best to check with your doctor first.

I'm worried that I might overdo things. Should I take any special precautions before exercising?

These are the guidelines.

- Don't exercise if you feel unwell, for instance if you've had flu or a bad cold. If you have had any recent illness, go back to exercising only when you have recovered and then build up slowly.

- If you get chest pain or breathing trouble while you are exercising, see your doctor.

- Don't exercise after a heavy meal or a hot bath – wait two to three hours before doing any.

- Avoid caffeine and alcohol for an hour before and after exercise.

Last time I tried jogging, I tore a calf muscle and was off work for 2 weeks. How can I avoid this happening again?

Don't exercise too hard too quickly and always loosen up first (see the warm-up exercises below) and do some cooling down exercises last: walk slowly for 3–5 minutes, stretch for 2 minutes. Never overdo it. One of the best things to do is to buy the correct shoes for the sport you are choosing (see question later regarding special clothing for exercising).

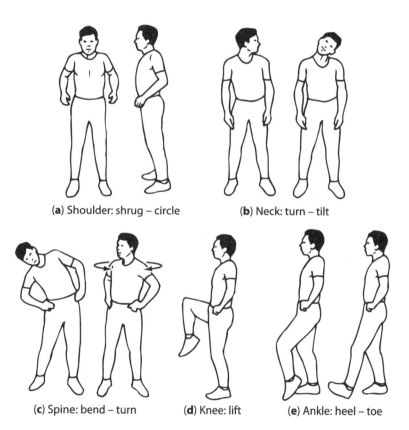

(**a**) Shoulder: shrug – circle   (**b**) Neck: turn – tilt

(**c**) Spine: bend – turn   (**d**) Knee: lift   (**e**) Ankle: heel – toe

CHOOSING YOUR EXERCISE

My local recreation centre offers 40 different sports from judo to meditation. What is the best form of exercise to do?

Any aerobic exercise is the best. This is dynamic exercise using large groups of muscles – for example walking, jogging, cycling and swimming. Non-aerobic exercise builds muscle strength (what is known as *isometrics*) but does little to help the heart's fitness and can be harmful, as it can make your blood pressure rise.

I lead a very busy life and just do not have time to exercise. Is there anything I can do?

Your health should always come first. No one on his death bed wished he'd spent more time at the office! However, you can exercise around your commitments.

- Climb the stairs rather than take the lift.
- Park so that you have to walk 200–300 yards to where you are going.
- If you use public transport, get off the bus, train, tram or tube a stop early and walk to or from the station.
- Walk the children to school.
- Take your young children to the park and run about with them.
- Clean you car rather than using the car-wash.

I am in my forties and have always hated competitive sport but enjoy walking. Is there a simple walking programme I could start?

Walking is especially good because it is cheap and generally safe and we all know how to do it. It also doesn't strain the joints as much as jogging or running. The American Heart Association walking programme (Table 10.2) is useful – but not compulsory – and you can vary the timing to your personal needs. 'Health Walks' are being developed by the Countryside Commission and the British Heart Foundation (see Appendix 2 for addresses).

You will need a yardstick to assess your progress. Try to find a distance of about one mile that you can walk; measure the distance by car or by striding out and counting the yards or metres. Alternatively, estimate the distance to the park, round the park or to the shops or station. If it's the shops, cancel the newspaper delivery and go each day to collect it.

- Gently loosen up by bending and stretching (Figure 10.1). Repeat exercises 1–5 up to six times before you start walking.

- Measure your heart rate by taking your pulse at the wrist or next to your Adam's apple. Count the number in 15 seconds and multiply by 4 or count the number in 6 seconds and add a 0. You now have the beats per minute (Figure 10.2).

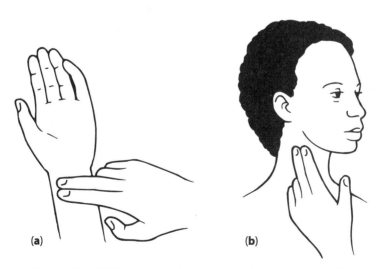

(a) (b)

Figure 10.2 Taking your pulse at your wrist (**a**) and neck (**b**).

- After walking for 5 minutes take your pulse again and speed up to get it above 110. If you are on a beta-blocker drug, this does not apply as these drugs slow the heart. Try to keep the pulse over 110 and note the time you took to complete your mile; take your pulse again whilst winding down. It should settle within 10 minutes.

Table 10.2 A simple walking programme

Weeks	Warm-up walking	Target zone walking*
Week 1		
Session A	5 min	briskly, 5 min
Session B	Repeat above pattern	
Session C	Repeat above pattern	

Continue with at least three exercise sessions during each week of the programme.

Week 2	5 min	briskly, 7 min
Week 3	5 min	briskly, 9 min
Week 4	5 min	briskly, 11 min
Week 5	5 min	briskly, 13 min
Week 6	5 min	briskly, 15 min
Week 7	5 min	briskly, 18 min
Week 8	5 min	briskly, 20 min
Week 9	5 min	briskly, 23 min
Week 10	5 min	briskly, 26 min
Week 11	5 min	briskly, 28 min
Week 12	5 min	briskly, 30 min

Week 13 on:
Check your pulse periodically to see if you are exercising within your target zone. As you become more fit, try exercising within the upper range of your target zone. Gradually increase your brisk walking time to 30–60 min, three or four times a week, Remember that your goal is to get the benefits that you are seeking and enjoy your activity.

---

* Your target zone is shown in Table 10.3.

- As you get fit, your walking time should shorten and your heart rate become slower and your recovery become quicker. You can then extend up to two miles, gradually increasing your walking speed and then your distance. Do not do too much too quickly.

Cool down walking	Total time
more slowly, 5 min	15 min
5 min	17 min
5 min	19 min
5 min	21 min
5 min	23 min
5 min	25 min
5 min	28 min
5 min	30 min
5 min	33 min
5 min	36 min
5 min	38 min
5 min	40 min

A friend of mine was told to judge his exercise by the talking test. What is this?

This is a simple but useful guide to how much exercise you are doing. You should be exercising in such a way that you can talk, but you should be a little breathless. If you can talk easily, you are not exercising briskly enough; if you cannot talk, you need to slow down.

I should like to go walking but I'm afraid to walk alone – I'm always reading in the local paper of women being attacked. Isn't it rather dangerous to walk on my own?

It is a sad reflection on the world that people, particularly women, should be afraid to go walking. Attacks do occur but are rare. We always need to keep a sense of proportion – only the bad things get reported. If, of 10 000 women walking in the countryside, only one was attacked, 9999 were not, but we would only hear of the one who suffered. Being afraid is understandable, but in the end it ruins your enjoyment of life. If you are worried, why not walk with two or three friends, or join a rambling club? Other precautions could include:

- carry an alarm or a mobile phone;
- do not go out when it's getting dark – pick the clear daylight hours;
- avoid remote areas and keep to open spaces (such as the paths in the park);
- choose the areas where there are lots of people (such as along a sea front or a popular park).

I've tried walking 1 mile a day and I find that I get bored after a month. What else can I do besides walking?

Joining a gym will give you access to a treadmill which will give you a better chance to judge your progress more accurately because of its computerised timing.

Other good exercises include rowing, swimming, cycling, dancing (aerobics) or simply climbing stairs. Variety is the thing!

There is a heart testing machine at my local gym, but frankly I do not understand what the figures mean. What should my maximum heart rate be?

Your maximum heart rate should be 220 minus your age. You should aim to get up to 75% of this. So, if you are aged 50, you should aim for three-quarters of 170, which is 127. When you begin your exercise programme, aim for 50% in the first 6–8 weeks and gradually build up to the 75%. Your target heart rate varies with age (see Table 10.3).

This guide applies to healthy people – those aiming to prevent heart disease. Those with heart disease should follow medical advice and limit activity based on awareness of breathing while still comfortable. Beta-blockers slow the heart rate for example, so using the pulse will not be

Table 10.3 Target heart rates

Age (years)	Target heart rate (bpm*)
20	100–150
30	95–142
40	90–135
50	85–127
60	80–120
70	75–113

* bpm: beats per minute

a good guide. Most people with heart problems can ignore the heart rate and exercise with the aim of progressively increasing performance.

I've got a tracksuit and trainers. Do I need any other special clothing to exercise in?

If you are going to build up a walking programme, you will need good shoes – don't cut corners in footwear. Walking or jogging shoes are the best, or proper walking boots if you are walking in the countryside. Wear thick socks when you try them on and look for shoes with cushion soles and an arch support. In warm weather, wear cool lightweight cotton and remember to put sunscreen skin cream on to guard against sunburn. In cooler weather, wear two or three layers (a vest, a T-shirt and a sweatshirt, for example) to retain the heat. Loose-fitting tracksuit bottoms are comfortable and inexpensive. Don't feel you have to go out in the rain – the exercise is to be enjoyed not endured.

Does regular exercise help prevent me from getting a heart attack during sex?

This is another good reason to get fit – physically fit people are sexually fit too and have far less risk of a heart problem during sex. Do you need another excuse?

What is 'exercise with a purpose'?

Some people need a reason for everything and can't see the point of just taking exercise – they get bored and lose interest. Exercise with a purpose gives them a reason, for example, walking to the newsagent for the daily paper, walking the dog, cleaning the car, getting off public transport early and walking the rest of the way to work and playing a sport such as tennis. All exercise like this is good for you. Remember alcohol in moderation is good for you, so walking as briskly as possible to and from the wine shop is exercise with a very good purpose!

| Glossary

AICD An automatic implantable cardioverter defibrillator, a type of pacemaker.

aneurysm Sac-like ballooning out of an artery wall, or scar tissue in the heart muscle.

angina Chest pain when the heart fails to get sufficient blood. Pain is usually a choking sensation which may spread to the jaw or arms.

angiography X-ray examination of the heart and coronary arteries. Under local anaesthetic, a catheter (fine tube) is passed to the heart and a dye shows up any narrowings or weaknesses. Also known as 'cardiac catheterisation'.

angioplasty Method of removing narrowings in arteries by the temporary insertion of a catheter with a tiny balloon on it. The balloon is inflated to squash the narrowing out of the way.

angiotensin converting enzyme (ACE) inhibitor Drug that lowers blood pressure and improves heart failure symptoms as well as life expectancy.

anticoagulant Drug that thins the blood (e.g. warfarin, heparin) and reduces its capacity to clot.

antioxidant Substance (e.g. vitamin C and E) which prevents fats becoming oxidised and thus allows the fats to build up on the arteries.

aorta Main artery which leaves the heart and runs down the back of the heart to the abdomen.

aortic valve Valve between the muscle pump on the left side of the heart (left ventricle) and the aorta.

arrhythmia Abnormal heartbeat.

artery Vessel carrying oxygen rich blood under pressure. Arterioles are small arteries.

atheroma (atherosclerosis) Fatty deposits on the lining of blood vessels (plaque).

atria Two upper chambers of the heart: left atrium and right atrium.

atrial fibrillation Chaotic heartbeats arising in the atria; always irregular.

atrial septal defect Hole in the heart between the right and left atria.

atrioventricular node Junction box in the electrical system of the heart, which helps prevent rapid heartbeats affecting the pump's action by limiting the number of beats that can get through.

automatic implantable cardioverter defibrillator *see* defibrillator

beta-blockers Drugs that block adrenaline thereby slowing the heart rate and lowering blood pressure. Used to treat angina, raised blood pressure, heart attacks and palpitations.

biopsy Removing a tissue sample.

blood clot Process where blood cells stick together like a jelly (or form a scab on the skin). It protects us from blood loss, but in the wrong place causes heart attacks.

blood pressure Pressure of the blood in the arteries.

blood vessels Tubes (arteries or veins) through which blood flows.

brachial artery Artery at the elbow used for blood pressure measurement.

bradycardia Slow heart rate (less than 60 beats per minute).

bundle branch block When one of the electric bundles in the heart is interrupted. There are two bundles, a right and left, and the block is described as right or left bundle branch block – abbreviated to RBBB or LBBB.

calcium antagonist (or **blocker**) Drugs that relax arteries by reducing calcium in the walls. Some also reduce irregular heartbeats. All lower blood pressure and help angina.

capillaries Smallest blood vessels joining arteries to veins.

cardiac Relating to the heart.

cardiac arrest A heart attack – when the heart suddenly stops beating and pumping blood.

cardiac catheter Fine tube threaded through an artery to the heart.

cardiac enzymes Enzymes looked for in a blood test to check for a heart attack.

cardiac output Amount of blood pumped by the heart each minute. Usually 5 litres.

cardiology Study of the heart in health and disease.

cardiologist Doctor specialising in heart disease – a physician not a surgeon.

cardiomyopathy Disease which weakens heart muscle.

cardiopulmonary bypass When a machine takes over the heart's work of pumping during surgery.

cardiovascular Relating to the heart and its blood vessels.

cardioversion Electric shock treatment for the heart, attempting to convert irregular rhythm to normal.

carotid arteries Main arteries running up both sides of the neck to the brain.

cerebral embolism Blood clot which has travelled to the brain.

cerebral haemorrhage Bleeding into the brain from a ruptured blood vessel.

cerebral thrombosis Blood clot blocking an artery to the brain.

cerebrovascular accident Death of brain tissue from a clot or a bleed.

cholesterol Fatty substance needed for cell building. Too much causes narrowed arteries. See also High density lipoprotein; Low density lipoprotein.

claudication Pain in the legs while walking caused by a lack of oxygen mainly from narrowed arteries – 'angina of the legs'.

collateral circulation ('collaterals') New small arteries which develop to bypass blocked ones.

conduction system Electrics of the heart.

congenital defects Heart problems (structural) that one is born with.

congestive heart failure *see* Heart failure

coronary arteries Arteries supplying blood to the heart.

coronary artery bypass graft (CABG) Surgery using veins or arteries to bypass narrowings or blockages in the coronary arteries.

coronary artery disease (CAD) Narrowing of the coronary arteries from fatty deposits.

coronary thrombosis Blood clot in a coronary artery usually leading to coronary artery narrowing.

deep-vein thrombosis (DVT) Clots in the veins of the leg.

defibrillator Equipment that delivers electric shocks to correct abnormal heartbeats.

diabetes Disease caused by lack of insulin, in which the body is unable to store sugar. May be treated with insulin, or diet and drugs.

diastole Relaxation of the heart between beats when it is filling with blood.

diastolic blood pressure (DBP) Lower of the two blood pressure readings taken when the heart is relaxing.

digoxin Drug used to strengthen the heart and control atrial fibrillation.

diuretic Water tablet that increases passage of fluid through the kidneys.

Doppler ultrasound Ultrasound technique used to study the speed and direction of blood flow. Sounds like a washing machine.

dyspnoea Shortness of breath.

echocardiography (echo) Painless means of studying the heart's structure by bouncing ultrasound waves off the heart.

ejection fraction (EF) Medical measure of the amount of blood pumped out of the left ventricle (pumping chamber) with each heartbeat, usually over 50%.

electrocardiogram (ECG or EKG) Recording of the electrical activity of the heart.

electrophysiological study (EPS) Catheter test to evaluate the source of irregular heartbeats and to judge the effect of treatments.

embolus Blood clot which travels in the circulation. Can be in the vein or artery.

endocarditis Infection inside the heart on a valve or the lining of the heart.

endothelium Smooth inner lining of an artery.

exercise test ('treadmill' test) ECG measures the heart's activity during exercise, usually on a treadmill. Used most often to diagnose coronary artery disease and assess its severity.

fatty acids Chemical parts of triglycerides.

fibrillation Erratic rapid contractions of the atria (atrial fibrillation) or ventricle (ventricular fibrillation). In ventricular fibrillation the heart stops.

fibrinogen Blood thickening agent which occurs naturally in the body.

flutter (atrial) A less erratic palpitation than atrial fibrillation.

free radicals Damaging molecules produced by normal body processes such as breathing (oxygen) and digestion. Antioxidants reduce their effects.

haemorrhage Bleeding.

heart attack Death of heart muscle from lack of blood supply.

heart block Slowing of the heart rate from an interrupted electrical circuit.

heart failure Known medically as congestive heart failure(CHF) or congestive **cardiac failure (CCF)** When the heart cannot meet the body's demands usually because of heart muscle weakness. See also Congestive heart failure.

heart-lung machine Machine that pumps blood to and from the body during heart surgery and keeps it full of oxygen.

heredity Inherited by genetic means.

hibernating myocardium Muscle which works but looks to be dead.

high blood pressure Serious increase in blood pressure.

high density lipoprotein (HDL) 'Good cholesterol' involved in removing cholesterol from the blood and blood vessels.

Holter monitor 24-hour ECG machine worn like a 'Walkman'.

hypercholesterolaemia High cholesterol in the blood.

hyperlipidaemia High fats in the blood.

hypertension High blood pressure.

hypotension Low blood pressure.

hypoxia Lack of oxygen.

ICD *see* AICD

immunosuppressive drugs Medication used to stop the body rejecting a transplant.

incompetence Valve that is leaking.

infarct Scar tissue with permanent damage to the heart muscle.

ischaemia Inadequate blood supply usually caused by narrowed arteries. Ischaemic heart disease (IHD) is the consequence of ischaemia from narrowed coronary arteries.

keloid Overgrowth of an operation scar.

lipids Fats.

lipoproteins Proteins, acting like taxis, carrying fats.

low density lipoprotein (LDL) 'Bad cholesterol' which sticks to the artery walls.

lumen Inside of a tube.

mitral valve Valve between the left atrium and left ventricle.

mitral valve prolapse (MVP) Floppy mitral valve causing one of the two leaflets to bulge backwards. This may cause a leak to occur but is often harmless.

monounsaturated fat Healthy sort of fat found in olive oil and peanut oil. Can lower LDL cholesterol.

mortality rate Number of deaths usually per year.

MRI *see* nuclear magnetic resonance

murmur Sound of blood flowing round, heard by a stethoscope. May be normal or point to disease. An echocardiogram will help diagnosis.

myocardial biopsy Taking a sample of heart muscle.

myocardial infarction (MI) Heart attack.

myocardial ischaemia Reduced (poor) blood supply to the heart muscle.

myocardium Heart muscle.

necrosis Death of body tissue.

nitroglycerin Drug used to relieve angina (e.g. glyceryl trinitrate – GTN).

non-invasive Means of diagnosis or treatment without the need for an incision.

nuclear magnetic resonance (NMR) Use of a magnetic field to take images of the heart and body. Also known as magnetic resonance imaging (MRI). NMR should not be undertaken if a pacemaker has been inserted but it can be used if a coronary stent is in place.

obesity Being overweight. Medical definition is 20% above the average for your height and weight.

occluded artery Totally blocked, may be acute or chronic.

oedema Fluid usually in the lungs or round the ankles.

open heart surgery Operation on the heart with the chest opened and a bypass machine used to pump the blood.

pacemaker Small electrical device implanted surgically that regulates the heartbeat usually preventing it going too slowly.

palpitations Out of the ordinary heartbeats. Can be rapid or missed or both.

passive smoking Breathing in (and being poisoned by) someone else's cigarette smoke.

Percutaneous coronary intervention (PCI) Angioplasty using either a balloon or a stent.

percutaneous transluminal coronary angioplasty (PTCA) Long-winded term for angioplasty.

pericarditis Inflammation of the pericardium.

pericardium Smooth sac that surrounds the heart. When inflamed, it loses smoothness and becomes painful, leading to pericarditis.

plaque Fatty deposits on the inner lining of an artery.

platelets Small blood particles which stick together to form clots. Aspirin reduces their stickiness.

polyunsaturated fat Fat in most vegetable oils which is liquid at room temperature. Tends to lower LDL cholesterol.

positron emission tomography (PET) Imaging technique that tells us whether the heart muscle is alive and how it is functioning. A very expensive technique, so used sparingly.

prophylaxis Anticipation and prevention, usually with drugs.

pulmonary Relating to the lungs and breathing system.

pulmonary valve Valve between the right ventricle and the pulmonary artery.

regurgitation Leaking, e.g. mitral regurgitation – a leaking mitral valve.

renal Relating to the kidneys.

resuscitation Reviving someone who seems to be dead by heart massage and mouth-to-mouth breathing.

risk factor Feature related to an increased chance of developing a disease (e.g. smoking and high cholesterol levels are risk factors for heart disease).

saturated fat Animal fat, solid at room temperature. Increases total and LDL cholesterol.

septum Muscle dividing the right from left side of the heart. A defect or hole in the heart is a 'septal defect'.

sestamibi scan The same procedure as a **thallium test**.

sinus node (sinoatrial or SA node) The heart's natural pacemaker or master switch.

sodium Sodium chloride is the chemical name for salt.

sphygmomanometer Machine to measure blood pressure.

stenosis Narrowing.

stent Meshwork tube inserted by a balloon into an artery, which, when expanded, holds an artery open. It is left in place. The balloon is removed.

sternum Breastbone.

stethoscope Instrument for listening to sounds in the body.

streptokinase Clot-dissolving drug.

stroke Damage to the brain as a result of interruption in the blood supply.

syncope Sudden loss of consciousness.

systole Heart contracting – pumping out blood.

systolic blood pressure Highest pressure measured when the heart contracts and pumps out blood.

tachycardia Rapid heartbeat, typically over 100 beats per minute.

thallium test Radioactive test to look at the extent of heart muscle damage (whether permanent or reversible).

thrombolysis Breaking down blood clots – 'clot busting'.

thrombosis Blood clot.

tissue plasminogen activator (TPA) Clot-dissolving treatment.

transoesophageal echocardiography (TOE) Specialised echo machine looking at the heart from inside the food pipe (oesophagus).

transplant Heart replaced with one from someone else.

triglycerides Fats used as energy source. High levels increase the risk for coronary disease.

unsaturated fats Fats that are liquid or a soft solid at room temperature.

vasodilator Drug that opens up (widens) arteries.

vein Low pressure blood vessels carrying blood back to the heart to pick up oxygen.

ventricle Heart muscle pump.

ventricular septal defect Hole between the right and left ventricle.

vitamin E Antioxidant vitamin found in vegetable oils, green leafy vegetables, wholegrain cereals, almonds and hazelnuts.

| Appendix 1

PRACTISING WHAT I PREACH

What do you do, as a doctor, to prevent heart disease?

With this question, people are really asking whether we, as doctors, follow our own advice. Not often, is the honest answer, but here is what I do. First, I have a family history of heart disease, so I'm more concerned with prevention as a result. This is very important.

- I don't smoke.

- I avoid salt and salty foods.

- I take regular exercise, walking briskly 2 miles a day, four times a week. I avoid lifts and take the stairs.

- I watch my weight. I eat sensibly but am not obsessed about it (see Chapter 9). I try to keep my cholesterol at 5.0 mmol/litre with a good HDL (see the section *Coronary artery disease and cholesterol* in Chapter 2).

- I enjoy wine.

- I have my blood pressure checked once a year.

- I try to stay calm!

What would you do if you had angina or a heart attack?

First, I would be disappointed that I had not been able to prevent it.

- I'd have my cholesterol checked again.

- I would take aspirin and medications prescribed.

- I would want to know how I did on an exercise test and how my pump performed on an echocardiogram.

What drugs would you take?

I would take aspirin, statin, ACE inhibitor or AII antagonists. I have mild asthma so I probably could not tolerate a beta-blocker.

Would you have an angiogram done?

I would not hesitate to have an angiogram or CT angiogram if this was recommended to determine the extent of the problem. I would want to look at it myself!

Would you have an angioplasty or surgery if recommended?

Again, I would have no hesitation in agreeing to whatever is appropriate. I would select my surgeon, cardiologist or anaesthetist carefully. I realise that I would have better information about this than a layman.

Would you return to your normal workload afterwards?

I would look carefully at my workload and almost certainly cut back on my commitments. I would try and reduce my hours, avoid committees and cut down on lectures and unnecessary travel. I would spend more time with my family, recognising that I should have done this much sooner. I would try to remember that no one on their deathbed wished they had spent more time at the office.

Do you think heart disease would affect you psychologically?

Yes. Like most doctors I have an unhealthy feeling of invincibility regarding my own health and it would shatter the myth! Being positive by nature would help me pick up the pieces, although I would have to recognise that those who 'told me so' were right.

| Appendix 2
Useful addresses and websites

If you write for information from any of these organisations, it is helpful to enclose a large self-addressed envelope. We have not included email numbers as these change frequently.

American College of Cardiology
Website: www.cardiosmart.org
A highly recommended website for information, articles and news.

American Heart Association
7272 Greenville Avenue
Dallas
Texas TX 75321
Tel: 00 1 800 242 8721
Fax: 00 1 214-706-2139
Website: www.americanheart.org
Promotes healthier life styles by training volunteers throughout the USA.

ASH (Action on Smoking and Health)
First Floor
144–145 Shoreditch High Street
London E1 6JE
Helpline: 0800 169 0169
Tel: 020 7739 5902
Fax: 020 7729 4732
Website: www.ash.org.uk
National organisation with local branches. Campaigns on antismoking policies. Offers free information on website or for sale from H.Q. Catalogue on request.

Blood Pressure Association
60 Cranmer Terrace
London SW17 0QS
Tel: 020 8772 4994
Fax: 020 8772 4999
Website: www.bpassoc.org.uk
Offers information and fact sheets about high blood pressure and the various ways it can be treated. An SAE A4 size envelope requested with two first class stamps.

British Acupuncture Council
63 Jeddo Road
London W12 9HQ
Tel: 020 8735 0400
Fax: 020 8735 0404
Website: www.acupuncture.org.uk
Professional body offering lists of qualified acupuncture therapists.

British Dietetic Association
5th Floor
Charles House
148–149 Great Charles Street
Birmingham B3 3HT
Tel: 0121 200 8080
Fax: 0121 200 8081
Website: www.bda.uk.com
Professional association supporting dietitians.

British Heart Foundation
14 Fitzhardinge Street
London W1H 4DH
Helpline: 08450 708070
Tel: 020 7935 0185
Fax: 020 7486 5820
Website: www.bhf.org.uk
Publications order line:
0870 600 6566
Funds research, promotes education and raises money to buy equipment to treat heart disease. HeartstartUK arranges training in emergency life-saving techniques. To contact local support groups tel. 020 7487 7110. The BHF also produces education materials. For information or to order a Publications and videos catalogue,

visit the website, or call the Publications orderline. You can download many of the publications from bhf.org.uk/publications free of charge, though a donation is welcome.

British Herbal Medicine Association
PO Box 583
Exeter EX1 9GX
Tel: 0845 680 1134
Fax: 0845 680 1136
Website: www.bhma.info
Offers information, encourages research and promotes high quality standards. Advises members on legalities for importers, vets advertisements and defends the right of the public to choose herbal medicines and be able to obtain them freely.

British Holistic Medical Association
PO Box 371
Bridgwater
Somerset TA6 9BG
Tel: 01278 722000
Website: www.bhma.org
Promotes awareness of the holistic approach to health among practitioners and the public through publications, self-help tapes, conferences and a network of local groups.

British Homeopathic Association
Hahnemann House
29 Park Street West
Luton LU1 3BE
Tel: 0870 444 3950
Fax: 0870 444 3960
Website: www.trusthomeopathy.org
Professional body offering lists of
qualified homeopathic practitioners.

British Hypertension Society
Clinical Sciences Building
Level 5
Leicester Royal Infirmary
PO Box 65
Leicester LE2 7LX
Tel: 07717 467 973
Website: www.bhsoc.org
Professional body disseminating
guidelines to health care professionals.

British Medical Acupuncture Society
BMAS House
3 Winningtom Court
Northwich
Cheshire CW8 1AG
Tel: 01606 786782
Fax: 01606 786783
Website: www.medical-acupuncture.co.uk
Professional body offering training to
doctors and list of accredited
acupuncture practitioners.

Cardiomyopathy Association
Unit 10, Chiltern Court
Asheridge Road
Chesham HP5 2PX
Tel: 01494 791224
Fax: 01494 797199
Website: www.cardiomyopathy.org
Offers information for health
professionals; also support and
information for people with
cardiomyopathy and their families.

Chest, Heart and Stroke Association (N. Ireland)
21 Dublin Road
Belfast BT2 7HB
Helpline: 08457 697 299
Tel: 02890 320 184
Fax: 02890 333 487
Website: www.nichsa.com
Funds research and provides
information on chest, heart and stroke-
related illnesses.

Chest, Heart and Stroke (Scotland)
65 North Castle Street
Edinburgh EH2 3LT
Helpline: 0845 077 6000
Tel: 0131 225 6963
Fax: 0131 220 6313
Website: www.chss.org.uk
Funds research and provides
information on chest, heart and
stroke-related illnesses.

Complementary Medical Association

Blackcleuch
Teviothead
Hawick
Scottish Borders TD9 0PU
Tel: 0845 129 8434
Website: www.the-cma.org.uk
A not-for-profit medical body offering membership to highly qualified practitioners of complementary medicine. Has a database of accredited practitioners around the UK.

Consumers' Association

2 Marylebone Road
London NW1 4DF
Helpline: 0845 307 4000
Tel: 020 7770 7000
Fax: 020 7770 7600
Website: www.which.net
Publications order line:
0800 252100.
Campaigns on behalf of consumers and produces reports on products including foods.

Coronary Prevention Group (CPG)

Website: www.healthnet.org.uk
First British charity devoted to prevention of coronary heart disease. Produces booklets and fact sheets available on the website or by post. Please send SAE.

Curative Hypnotherapy Register

584 Adams Hill
Derby Road
Nottingham NG7 2GZ
Tel: 0115 970 1233
Website:
www.curativehypnotherapyregister.co.uk
Professional membership body, offers information about hypnotherapy and a list of registered practitioners.

Department of Health (DoH)

PO Box 777
London SE1 6XH
Helpline: 0800 555 777
Tel: 020 7210 4850
Fax: 01623 724 524
Textphone: 020 7210 5025
Website: www.doh.gov.uk
Produces literature about health issues, available via helpline. A more technical site with National Service Frameworks available from Internet e.g. www.doh.gov.uk/nsf/bloodpressure

Diabetes UK

10 Parkway
London NW1 7AA
Helpline: 020 7424 1030
Tel: 020 7424 1000
Textline 020 7424 1031
Fax: 020 7424 1001
Website: www.diabetes.org.uk
Provides advice and information on diabetes; has local support groups.

Drinkline (National Alcohol Helpline)
Helpline: 0800 917 8282
Funded by Dept. of Health, provides educational material for schools, health professionals and general information on drink, sex and drugs issues. Refers to local agencies for support.

Health Development Agency
Holborn Gate
330 High Holborn
London WC1V 7BA
Helpline: 0870 121 4194
Tel: 020 7430 0850
Fax: 020 7061 3390
Website: www.hda-online.org.uk
Formerly Health Education Authority; now only deals with research. Publications on health matters can be ordered on 0800 555 777.

Health Which?
PO Box 44
Hertford X SG14 1LH
Tel: 0800 252100
Fax: 0845 3074001
Website: www.which.net
Requests for any Consumer Association (Which?) publications, can be ordered here.

Heart UK
7 North Road
Maidenhead SL6 1PE
Tel: 01628 628 638
Fax: 01628 628 698
Website: www.heartuk.org.uk
Offers information, advice and support to people with coronary heart disease and especially to those at high risk of familial hyper- cholesterolaemia. Members receive bimonthly magazine.

Institute for Complementary Medicine
Can-Mezzanine
32–36 Loman Street
London SE1 0EH
Tel: 020 922 7980
Fax: 020 922 7981
Website: www.icmedicine.co.uk
Umbrella group for complementary medicine organisations. Offers informed, safe choice to public, British register of practitioners and refers to accredited training courses. S.a.e. requested for information.

Irish Heart Foundation
4 Clyde Road
Ballsbridge
Dublin 4
Tel: 00 353 1 668 5001
Fax: 00 353 1 668 5896
Website: www.irishheart.ie
*Offers information, publications,
training and support in prevention of
heart disease. Collaborates with other
heart-related organisations and has
some local support groups.*

**National Institute
of Medical Herbalists**
Elm House
54 Mary Arches Street
Exeter EX4 3BA
Tel: 01392 426 022
Fax: 01392 498 963
Website: www.nimh.org.uk
*Professional body representing
qualified, practising medical
herbalists. Offer lists of accredited
medical herbalists. S.A.E. requested.*

Natural England
(formerly Countryside Agency)
Northminster House
Peterborough PE1 1UA
Tel: 0845 600 3078
Fax: 01733 455103
Website: www.countryside.gov.uk
*Working with other agencies,
identifies problems and develops
solutions to economic, environmental
and community issues for the
enjoyment of the countryside.*

**NHS Direct (England,
Northern Ireland & Wales)**
Helpline: 0845 4647
Tel: 020 8867 1367
Textphone 0845 606 4647
Website: www.nhsdirect.nhs.uk
*NHS Direct is a 24 hour helpline
offering confidential healthcare advice,
information and referral service 365
days of the year. A good first port of
call for any health advice.*

NHS Health Scotland
Woodburn House
Canaan Lane
Edinburgh EH10 4SG
Tel: 0131 536 5500
Fax: 0131 536 5501
Textphone 0131 536 5503
Website: www.healthscotland.com
NHS Scotland 0800 224 488
*NHS health education board for
Scotland publishing leaflets on a
variety of health issues.*

Quit (National Society for Non-Smokers)
211 Old Street
London EC1V 9NR
Helpline: 0800 002200
Tel: 020 7251 1551
Fax: 020 7251 1661
Website: www.quit.org.uk
Offers advice to stop smoking in English and Asian languages; also to schools, and on pregnancy. Runs training courses for health professionals. Can put people in touch with local support groups.

Resuscitation Council
5th Floor, Tavistock House North
Tavistock Square
London WC1H 9HR
Tel: 020 7388 4678
Fax: 020 7383 0773
Website: www.resus.org.uk
Sets standards and runs courses on resuscitation for health care professionals. Funds research.

Royal Life Saving Society UK
River House, High Street
Broom B50 4HN
Tel: 01789 773994
Fax: 01789 773995
Website: www.lifesavers.org.uk
Leading organisation promoting prevention of drowning through training and activities in life-saving techniques.

Scottish Heart and Arterial Disease Risk Prevention (SHARP)
Department of Medicine
and Therapeutics
Ninewells Hospital and Medical School
Dundee DD1 9SY
Tel: 01382 660111
Fax: 01382 660675
Website: www.heartscotland.org
Charity run by health professionals aiming, through scientific meetings and research, to reduce incidence of cardiovascular disease in Scotland. Produces guidelines for health professionals, leaflets and videos for their patients.

Sexual Dysfunction Association
Suite 301, Emblem House
London Bridge Hospital
27 Tooley Street
London SE1 2PR
Helpline: 0870 7743571
(Monday, Wednesday, Friday 10 am–4 pm)
Website: www.sda.uk.net
Gives advice on sexual problems, such as erectile dysfunction.

Smoking
Two good websites to help you stop smoking are
www.giveupsmoking.co.uk
www.bhf.org.uk/smoking

Society of Homeopaths
11 Brookfield
Duncan Close
Moulton Park
Northampton NN3 6WL
Tel: 0845 450 6611
Fax: 0845 450 6622
Website: www.homeopathy-soh.org
*Professional body, offers lists of
accredited homeopathic therapists and
free general information.*

Sport England
3rd Floor
Victoria House
Bloomsbury Square
London WC1B 4SE
Tel: 020 7273 1551
Fax: 020 7383 5740
Website: www.sportengland.org
*Government agency promoting sport
in England with a wide variety of
activity programmes in order to foster
a healthier lifestyle.*

St John Ambulance
27 St John's Lane
London EC1M 4BU
Helpline: 08700 104 950
Tel: 020 7324 4000
Fax: 020 7324 4001
Website: www.sja.org.uk
*Provides first aid training for adults
and young people and cover for events.
Has a fleet of ambulances and provides
services to homeless people and library
services to hospitals.*

Stroke Association
Stroke House
240 City Road
London EC1V 2PR
Helpline: 0845 303 3100
Tel: 020 7566 0300
Fax: 020 7490 2686
Textphone: 020 7251 9096
Website: www.stroke.org.uk
*Funds research and provides
information now specialising in stroke
only. Publications can be ordered from
01604 623 933.*

**Vegetarian Society
of the United Kingdom**
Parkdale
Dunham Road
Altrincham WA14 4QG
Tel: 0161 925 2000
Fax: 0161 926 9182
Website: www.vegsoc.org
*Offers information on the vegetarian
way of life, day and residential
training courses at own Centre.
Provides literature for GCSE projects,
advice to school caterers. Food
manufacturers and restaurants can
apply for vegetarian accreditation.*

Women's Health Concern (WHC)
4–6 Eton Place
Marlow SL7 2QA
Helpline: 0845 123 2319
Tel: 01628 478 473
Fax: 01628 482 743
Website: www.womens-health-concern.org
National charity that offers help to
women, particularly on questions of
hormone health, HRT and
gynaecology. Request S.A.E. for
information. Website for menopause
queries: www.menopausematters.co.uk

| Appendix 3
Useful publications

Books

High Blood Pressure: Answers at your fingertips, by Dr Tom Fahey, Professor Deirdre Murphy with Dr Julian Tudor Hart, published by Class Publishing (2004). ISBN 978 1 85959 090 4

Type 2 Diabetes: Answers at your fingertips, by Dr Charles Fox and Dr Anne Kilvert, published by Class Publishing (2007). ISBN 978 1 85959 176 5

Dump Your Toxic Waist! by Dr Derrick Cutting, published by Class Publishing (2008). ISBN 978 1 85959 191 8

30 Minutes a Day to a Healthy Heart, published by Readers Digest (2006). ISBN 978 0 27644 065 6

General booklets

The **British Heart Foundation** publishes many excellent and recently revised booklets on all aspects of heart disease, including Women and heart disease; Smoking and your heart; Implantable cardioverter defibrillators; Trim the fat from your diet; Put your heart into walking. Head office and regional addresses can be found in Appendix 2.

In Scotland, the **SHARP programme** is an excellent source of information – information is available online at www.dundee.ac.uk/sharp/

The Family Doctor Series covers around 27 titles including cholesterol, stress and high blood pressure; individual booklets are priced very cheaply. Published by FDP, PO Box 4664, Poole BH15 1NN, Tel: 01202 668330

Ask your doctor for free leaflets that may have been provided by drug companies, and also from local NHS Trusts etc.

The **Coronary Prevention Group** (address in Appendix 2) provides good advice. Look on their website for further information.

Diabetes UK publishes a leaflet on Eating well with diabetes, which should be useful for people with diabetes and heart problems.

In America, it is difficult to beat the booklets from the **American Heart Association** (address in Appendix 2). Website address: www.americanheart.org – many publications listed are listed on their website, including To Your Health! A Guide to Heart-Smart Living; Fitting in Fitness; 365 Ways to Get Out the Fat: A Tip a Day to Trim the Fat Away and 6 Weeks to Get Out the FAT.

Food and cooking

Cooking for a healthy heart by Jacqui Lynas, published by Hamlyn/Heart UK (2004). ISBN 0 600610 51 9

Healthy Heart: Best-Kept Secrets of the Women's Institute, by Elspeth Smith, published by Simon & Schuster (2005). ISBN 0 743 25978 5

Stopping smoking

How to Stop Smoking and Stay Stopped for Good, by Gillian Riley, published by Vermilion (2007). ISBN 978 0 0919 1703 6

Stop Smoking in Five Days by Judy Perlmutter, published by HarperCollins (1997). ISBN 0 722535 83 X

Allen Carr's Easy Way to Stop Smoking, by Allen Carr, published by Penguin (2006). ISBN 978 0 1410 2689 3

| Appendix 4
Guideline desirable weight in adults

	Height in flat shoes		Average weight in pounds and kilograms (in indoor clothing)								
			17–19 yr			20–24 yr			25–29 yr		
	cm	ft in	kg	st	lb	kg	st	lb	kg	st	lb
MEN	157.5	5 2	54.0	8	7	58.1	9	0	60.8	9	7
	160.0	5 3	55.8	8	11	59.9	9	6	62.6	9	11
	162.6	5 4	57.6	9	1	61.7	9	10	64.0	10	1
	165.1	5 5	59.4	9	4	63.0	9	13	65.3	10	4
	167.6	5 6	61.2	9	8	64.4	10	1	67.1	10	7
	170.2	5 7	63.0	9	13	65.8	10	4	68.5	10	11
	172.7	5 8	64.9	10	3	67.6	10	8	70.3	11	1
	175.3	5 9	66.7	10	7	69.4	10	13	72.1	11	4
	177.8	5 10	68.5	10	11	71.2	11	3	73.9	11	8
	180.3	5 11	70.3	11	1	73.0	11	7	75.8	11	13
	182.9	6 0	72.6	11	6	75.3	11	11	78.0	12	4
	185.4	6 1	74.4	11	10	77.1	12	1	80.3	12	8
	188.0	6 2	76.2	12	0	78.9	12	6	82.6	13	0
	190.5	6 3	78.0	12	4	80.8	12	10	84.4	13	4
	193.0	6 4	79.8	12	8	82.1	12	13	86.2	13	8
WOMEN	147.3	4 10	44.9	7	1	46.3	7	4	48.5	7	8
	149.9	4 11	46.3	7	4	47.6	7	7	49.9	7	11
	152.4	5 0	47.6	7	7	49.0	7	10	51.3	8	1
	154.9	5 1	49.4	7	11	50.8	8	0	52.6	8	4
	157.5	5 2	51.3	8	1	52.2	8	3	54.0	8	7
	160.0	5 3	52.6	8	4	53.5	8	6	55.3	8	10
	162.6	5 4	54.4	8	8	54.9	8	8	56.7	8	13
	165.1	5 5	56.2	8	11	56.7	8	13	58.5	9	3
	167.6	5 6	57.6	9	1	58.5	9	3	60.3	9	7
	170.2	5 7	59.0	9	4	59.9	9	6	61.7	9	10
	172.7	5 8	60.8	9	7	61.7	9	10	63.5	10	0
	175.3	5 9	62.6	9	11	63.5	10	0	65.3	10	4
	177.8	5 10	64.4	10	1	65.3	10	4	67.1	10	7
	180.3	5 11	66.7	10	7	67.6	10	8	69.4	10	13
	182.9	6 0	68.9	10	11	69.9	11	0	71.7	11	4

This is just a guide. A more accurate assessment is provided in Figure 9.1.

Average weight in pounds and kilograms (in indoor clothing)											
30–39 yr			40–49 yr			50–59 yr			60–69yr		
kg	st	lb	kg	st	lb	kg	st	lb	kg	st	lb
62.1	9	11	63.5	10	0	64.4	10	1	63.0	9	13
64.0	10	1	65.3	10	4	65.8	10	4	64.4	10	1
65.8	10	4	67.1	10	8	67.6	10	8	66.2	10	6
67.6	10	8	68.9	10	11	69.4	10	13	68.0	10	10
69.4	10	13	70.8	11	1	71.2	11	3	69.9	11	0
71.2	11	3	73.0	11	7	73.5	11	8	72.1	11	4
73.0	11	7	74.8	11	11	75.3	11	11	73.9	11	8
74.8	11	11	76.7	12	1	77.1	12	1	76.2	12	0
77.1	12	1	78.9	12	6	79.4	12	7	78.5	12	4
78.9	12	6	80.8	12	10	81.6	12	11	80.8	12	7
81.2	12	11	83.0	13	1	83.9	13	3	83.0	13	1
83.0	13	1	84.8	13	4	85.7	13	7	85.3	13	6
85.3	13	6	87.1	13	10	88.0	13	11	87.5	13	11
87.5	13	11	89.4	14	1	90.3	14	3	89.8	14	1
90.3	14	3	92.1	14	7	93.0	14	8	92.5	14	7
52.2	8	3	55.3	8	10	56.7	8	13	57.6	9	1
53.1	8	4	56.2	8	11	57.6	9	1	58.5	9	3
54.4	8	7	57.6	9	1	59.0	9	4	59.4	9	4
55.8	8	11	59.0	9	4	60.3	9	7	60.8	9	7
57.2	9	0	60.3	9	7	61.7	9	10	62.1	9	11
58.5	9	3	61.7	9	10	63.5	10	0	64.0	10	1
59.9	9	6	63.5	10	0	65.3	10	4	65.8	10	4
61.2	9	8	64.9	10	3	67.1	10	8	67.6	10	8
63.0	9	13	66.7	10	7	68.9	10	11	69.4	10	13
64.4	10	1	68.5	10	11	70.8	11	4	71.2	11	3
66.2	10	6	70.3	11	1	72.6	11	6	73.0	11	7
68.0	10	10	72.1	11	4	74.4	11	10	74.8	11	11
69.9	11	0	74.4	11	10	76.7	12	1	–	–	
72.1	11	4	76.7	12	1	78.9	12	6	–	–	
74.4	11	10	78.9	12	6	81.6	12	11	–	–	

| Index